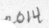

The Plan

P*the*lan

Eliminate the Surprising
"Healthy" Foods That
Are Making You Fat—
and Lose Weight Fast

LYN-GENET RECITAS

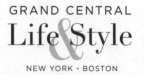

GRAND CENTRAL
Life&Style
NEW YORK · BOSTON

Grand Central Life & Style
Hachette Book Group
1290 Avenue of the Americas
New York, NY 10104

www.GrandCentralLifeandStyle.com

Printed in the United States of America

RRD-C

First trade edition: December 2014
10 9 8 7 6 5 4 3 2 1

Grand Central Life & Style is an imprint of Grand Central Publishing. The Grand Central Life & Style name and logo are trademarks of Hachette Book Group, Inc.

The Hachette Speakers Bureau provides a wide range of authors for speaking events. To find out more, go to www.HachetteSpeakersBureau.com or call (866) 376-6591.

The publisher is not responsible for websites (or their content) that are not owned by the publisher.

The Library of Congress has cataloged the hardcover edition as follows:
Recitas, Lyn-Genet.
    The plan : eliminate the surprising "healthy" foods that are making you fat—and lose weight fast / by Lyn-Genet Recitas. —First edition.
        pages ; cm
    Includes index.
    ISBN 978-1-4555-1548-6 (hardcover)—ISBN 978-1-4555-1549-3 (trade pbk.)—ISBN 978-1-4555-1550-9 (ebook)   1. Weight-loss—Health aspects. 2. Body weight—Health aspects.   3. Nutrition—Physiology.   I. Title.
    RM222.2.R424 2013
    613.2'5—dc23

                                                                    2012033716

Contents

Introduction

You've tried diet after diet.

You eat well.

You exercise.

Yet you're still gaining weight. Maybe a little, maybe a lot. Or maybe you're not gaining, but you just can't seem to drop those unwanted pounds the way you used to. At the same time, you might suffer from hormonal disorders, migraines, depression, skin conditions, joint pain, IBS, Crohn's, or other ailments. One day you step on the scale after eating healthy foods and your weight is up, and you have no idea why. You get frustrated and spend the next day eating cookies, and your weight stabilizes. You start to wonder if you should go on the cookie diet and at least have fun! You've tried everything that used to work: dieting, juice fasts, exercise—and still the weight isn't budging. If you're anything like the thousands of people I've worked with, you're seriously frustrated.

Why isn't your body responding??

It's pretty simple, actually. Your weight is nothing more than a reflection of your body's chemical reaction to foods. I want you to pause for a second here and repeat that out loud (yes, really): *Weight gain is nothing more than my body's chemical reaction to foods.* You're not eating too many carbs, or too much fat, or too many calories. You're simply eating certain reactive foods that are triggering an inflammatory response. And when your body is rife with inflammatory chemicals, it can cause a whole host of problems. Weight gain, migraines, skin conditions, high blood pressure—low-grade inflammation is the culprit behind all of them, aided and abetted by reactive foods that appear so righteous on the surface but are steadily and sneakily making us overweight, depressed, and sick.

And yes, I'm talking about supposedly healthy foods like oatmeal, salmon, turkey, beans, Greek yogurt, and more. That's why you're frustrated, my dear friend—and understandably so! All those things you've been told for years are "good for you" are actually the problem, insidiously packing on the pounds and sapping your health and vitality while you suffer and deprive yourself.

It's hard to believe, but cookies and nachos are not the problem. We know if we overdo it on junk day in and day out we'll gain weight. That's not a surprise. You don't eat them and say, "Wow, why didn't I lose weight and feel vitally healthy?" You do it because it's fun, and you should be able to indulge occasionally. But fish? Green beans? Tomato sauce? If you spend the day eating cupcakes and gain a pound, well, okay. Maybe you go to the gym the next day and it's gone. But if you spend a day eating healthy foods and you gain a pound, there's a problem. And I'm going to help you find it.

Your body is constantly communicating with you about what foods do and do not work for it in ways you might not be aware of: fatigue, poor stress response, digestive issues—these are all signals that your body is sending as an alert to please stop eating that food. But how do you know which foods? How do you interpret the signals? I'm here to help you put all the pieces of the puzzle together.

Welcome to The Plan. The next twenty days are going to be a controlled experiment to help you discover which foods do and don't work for your body. Every person's chemistry is unique, and we're going to systematically test foods to learn how *your* body reacts, so you can start making informed choices.

The Plan is divided into three phases. Phase One, the Three-Day

Cleanse, will be an easy detox to create a neutral base line in your body. In Phase Two, the Testing Phase (Days Four through Twenty), we're going to test specific foods and your favorite restaurants as we home in on your "friendly" or "reactive" foods. Don't worry; if a food you love turns out to be reactive for you, it doesn't mean it's banished from your life forever. You'll learn how to easily work it in and enjoy it in an informed way. After that, in Phase Three, Testing on Your Own, you'll learn how to create your own menus and tests and analyze your body's responses, so that The Plan becomes a natural and easy way of life.

By the time we're done, you'll see an average weight loss of up to 8 percent of your body weight and a dramatic improvement in sleep patterns, energy level, digestive function, and wellness (many clients are able to wean themselves off medications they've been taking for years). All of these things happen when we root out your reactive foods, which cause inflammation, and allow the body to do what it most wants to do, which is repair, renew, and balance. Most of all, you'll be armed with invaluable knowledge of how your body processes different foods so you'll never again get sideswiped by mystery weight gain or symptoms that appear seemingly out of nowhere.

The Plan is not a diet program. I don't want you to eat macrobiotic, or vegan, or low-fat, or low-carb, or whatever other kind of regimen you've followed in the past. I want you to discover your own particular hidden saboteurs so you can eat like you, according to what works for your particular body. This is about creating *your* plan. It's not *my* plan. Okay, yes, it starts out as "The Plan," and yes, there's protocol you need to follow for these twenty days. But the ultimate goal is to empower you to create your own personalized plan, which will change your relationship to food not just for these twenty days, but for the rest of your life.

Here's just some of what you'll discover on The Plan:

- Why the foods we think are the problem aren't the problem. I can't tell you how many people are *gaining* weight snacking on celery sticks and hummus when they could be eating potato chips and guacamole and *losing* weight.

- Which are your "friendly" foods, and which are your "reactive" foods. (Note that I didn't say "good" or "bad"—there are no good or bad foods, only the foods that work, and don't work, for your body.)

- Why the very thing you've come to hate—the scale—is your new best friend. Your daily weight is nothing more than data, and we're going to use this data to inform you how your body is reacting to certain foods. You'll come to appreciate your scale as a highly useful interpretive device!

- How to determine whether your thyroid is sluggish (even if it tested normal) and is sabotaging your weight loss efforts, and how to easily reverse that.

- How you can enjoy the foods you love most and still lose weight and feel fantastic.

- How to create delicious menus that will help you maintain your weight and meet your health goals for the rest of your life.

Within twenty days, you will be well on your way to reaching your goals of eating healthier, awaking refreshed and energized, and, of course, losing weight. No more feeling tyrannized and confused. Most of all, no deprivation. I want to bring the joy of eating back into your life. I love good food! I come from a long career in the restaurant business and spent years immersed in the world of wonderful food like great steaks, cheeses, desserts, and, of course, lots of good wine. Those things are still very much part of my life, and if you love them, there's a good chance they'll be part of yours, too. I want you to stop having to avoid "fun" food and understand that you shouldn't put the kibosh on that steak served with bread and butter— it might very well be better for you than an egg-white omelet.

We've become so fearful of foods, hearing conflicting advice of "don't eat this" and "don't eat that," that we think we can only order a salad when we go out. Look, anyone can lose weight by limiting themselves to 500 or 800 calories a day. But that's no way to live! I want you to understand that all the information you read and all the diets you've been on are a compilation of averages. If something works for 70 percent of the population, it's considered highly effective. But what if you're among the other 30 percent?

Plus, where's the joy in denying yourself good food? It's depressing to feel like you can't go out and enjoy a wonderful meal. If I suggested a handful of foods that were universally "Plan friendly" that my clients were restricted to, I'd have a lot of very unhappy people on my hands. I want you to be able to stay on The Plan for the rest of your life, and that includes eating out and enjoying yourself. The Plan will empower you wherever you are—at home, in a restaurant, at a party, even on vacation. You'll have peace of mind, knowing how to choose the foods (even decadent ones) that give you joy and glowing health and that work with your unique body to make you look and feel strong, sexy, lean, and beautiful.

This is an important life change you're about to embark on. It requires work, but if you solidly commit yourself for at least ten days, we can get the basics. If you commit for the full twenty, we'll change your life. I am so happy to be on this journey with you.

Lyn-Genet Recitas

Part One

UNLOCKING THE WEIGHT GAIN MYSTERY

CHAPTER ONE

What's Going Wrong?

Carolyn, forty-four, came to me in a state of desperation. She'd tried every diet, cleanse, and pill to lose the twenty pounds that had slowly but steadily crept on over the past few years, with no results. She ate well and exercised four times a week but still felt sluggish and depressed most of the time. She'd been to the top doctors, diet gurus, boot camps, and more, searching for solutions, but everyone gave her conflicting advice, which confused her even further. By the time she called me, she was living on Zoloft, caffeine, and 800 calories a day, but the heaviness in her mind and around her waistline wasn't budging.

Jonathan, fifty-one, was aggravated. He couldn't lose the forty pounds that plagued him, even though he stuck to "perfect" diet foods like oatmeal, salads, and grilled salmon. Even more upsetting to Jonathan was the gout and high cholesterol that he couldn't seem to get under control. He was doing everything "right," but nothing was working.

Thirty-eight-year-old Jessica's experience was not as severe but was just as frustrating. "I never know what size I'm going to be on any given day," she sighed. "One day my jeans fit completely fine, and the next I can't even zip them because I'm so bloated. I can go for days with my stomach distended and I have no idea why, and then out of nowhere it's flat again. I feel like I have no control over my own body."

I've worked with thousands of clients like Carolyn, Jonathan, and Jessica: women and men who don't know what to eat anymore because it seems like everything makes them gain weight; who have conflated every diet plan they've ever tried and are down to only five foods in their rotation; who feel tired, depressed, or bloated, or suffer from IBS, chronic pain, constipation, eczema, and other maladies that are making them miserable.

These are smart, health-savvy people we're talking about. They've tried everything that *should* work, with no results. Eating clean, exercise, even extreme cleanses or detox diets that might have sloughed off the pounds in the past suddenly aren't making a bit of difference. The less things make sense, the more people come to distrust their bodies. And frankly, that's a bad place to be.

It's time to cut through all the diet hype and solve this perplexing mystery once and for all. We're going to get to the bottom of what's actually causing your weight gain and other painful or even debilitating symptoms. I promise, your body isn't betraying you, even though it feels that way. And food isn't the enemy. Absolutely not! Good food can nourish us physically and emotionally, just like diets can starve our bodies and spirits. No, neither your body nor food is the enemy here. Misinformation is. What's going wrong, very simply, is that we have the wrong information about what it really takes to lose weight.

Here are the "basics" that most of us have been taught to believe:

- There are healthy foods and bad foods. Stick to the healthy foods and you'll stay slim and vibrant.
- Eating in moderation is the key to weight loss.
- Fats should be kept to a minimum.
- If you burn more calories than you consume, you'll lose weight.
- Women should stick to 1,500 calories per day for weight loss, men to 1,800.

But what if you're doing everything "right" and still gaining weight or dealing with persistent health issues? Why are we gaining weight from seemingly healthy foods like turkey and asparagus—and why are our health issues cropping up when we do? There's more to the story here, my dear friends, and I'm here to tell you what it is.

Talia, 35

If anyone has ever doubted that they could lose weight in a healthy way and actually be able to maintain the loss, then they must try The Plan. I have gone through my good share of diets but always struggled with how to permanently keep the weight off without depriving my body of the nutrients it needs.

I initially came to Lyn because I wanted to lose a few pounds and figure out why I always felt bloated after meals. While on The Plan, I lost twenty pounds in two months and began to develop a conceptual understanding of the way my body digests and processes foods. I was no longer feeling bloated and overall felt more energized and healthy.

The best part is I have been able to maintain my weight and still feel as great today as I did when I started The Plan. One of the immediate results I noticed was how much my relationship ·to food changed. My cravings for certain "unhealthy" foods diminished. I gained new knowledge of what "friendly foods" vs "highly reactive foods" were for me. As a result, I went from not cooking to making regular family dinners, grocery shopping, studying nutrition labels, and learning how to pick out the right foods for myself. I started making healthier choices when I was eating out and was no longer feeling guilty about meals I was ordering. I never felt like I was depriving myself of good food. In fact, on the occasions when I would splurge and "go off The Plan" for an evening, I knew exactly what to do to lose the one to three pounds I might have gained.

Doing The Plan is so much more than just losing weight. It transforms your relationship to food in the most positive way imaginable. When people ask me "What diet did you do?" I get confused. My response always is "I didn't go on a diet. I just figured out what foods were right for my body." And that's the great advantage of it; you're not dieting—you're revolutionizing the way you eat for the rest of your life and changing the way you feel on the inside and out.

The Insidious Offender: Inflammation

The hidden culprit behind all of this is inflammation. The idea that low-grade inflammation is behind nearly every disease and ailment has moved to the front burner within the medical community over the past decades. Countless studies have linked chronic low-grade inflammation to cancer, diabetes, heart disease, IBS, Crohn's, Alzheimer's, Parkinson's, polycystic ovarian syndrome (PCOS), infertility, premature aging, and obesity. Medical journals publish article after article about the dangerous effects of chronic inflammation, and now the mainstream media has caught on. In 2004, *Time* magazine ran a cover story labeling inflammation "The Silent Killer." Bestselling authors and health gurus Dr. Andrew Weil and Dr. Mark Hyman have written books about the connection between inflammation, aging, health, and weight loss. *Allure*, *Harper's Bazaar*, and *Vogue* magazines have all run articles about how inflammation attacks the body from a cosmetic and health perspective.

In its primary function, inflammation is a good thing. It's the body's immunologic response to an injury or illness that allows us to fight off infection. We want our inflammatory response to kick in when we injure ourselves, to speed the healing process and help protect our tissues. The problems occur when the inflammation doesn't subside and becomes chronic in our system. When the body is rife with inflammatory chemicals, our latent health issues get triggered, we age prematurely, and yes—we gain weight.

Most doctors shrug their shoulders at this, but the foods you choose can actually hasten or reverse the inflammatory process. We all have certain foods that are inflammatory for us. These foods might be healthy in a vacuum, but when combined with our body's unique chemistry, they can be quite toxic. When we eat one of these trigger foods, our bodies, being the brilliant machines they are, sense that something toxic has been introduced into our system. The body goes on high alert, thinking it is under attack, and it floods the tissues with water, trying to keep that toxic substance (and the hormones and chemicals it has released) away from the brain and other vital tissues—enter swelling, rashes, itching, and tissue damage. As the body continues to divert all its energy to the problem, other body systems start to slow down as a result, including digestion, circulation, and cognitive function (hello, weight gain, joint pain, depression...). In addition, 60 to 70 percent of your immune system is located in your gut-associated lymphatic tissue (known as GALT), so when you impair digestion, guess what happens to your health response? Until your body is able to excrete the perceived toxin, it's in your system doing its dirty work. This reaction to food can easily last 72 hours.

Weight gain is nothing more than your body's chemical reaction to certain foods. You eat something that is reactive for you, an inflammatory response is triggered, your digestion is impaired, and suddenly you're up a pound or two. The mistake would be in stopping there and saying that salmon or popcorn or whatever else causes weight gain. It's never the food itself that causes weight gain. It's the chemical response it triggers in your body that makes the number on the scale tick upward and awakens latent health issues.

Whenever you see a pound or more of weight gain, you'll see a corresponding health response—even if you're not consciously aware of it as a problem. I always have clients fill out an intake questionnaire about their goals and any health issues they have, and about 60 percent of them say they have no health issues. But then they start going through The Plan and suddenly realize that those under-eye bags are gone, they're sleeping through the night, or they can walk up two flights of stairs without their knees aching. Those symptoms that they always thought were "normal" are actually anything but.

And it's not just physical symptoms we're talking about. So many of us lead stressful lives, and we beat ourselves up for not being in better control of our emotions. But food has a great deal to do with that, too. Reactive foods can cause depression and poor stress responses and affect cognitive function. Most people don't even see it, like my client Angela, age forty-one, who was a stressed-out mom of two young kids. She beat herself up a lot for having such a short fuse with them, but she didn't realize that it was specific foods that were making her react. We started to identify her trigger foods, and sure enough, she came to see that within ten minutes of consuming one of these foods, she'd be screaming at her kids. And then her weight would be up the next day as well. Anytime you're not operating at your best—whether it's mentally, physically, or emotionally—there's an underlying reason for it, and very often it's a reactive food.

Remove reactive foods and a wonderful thing happens. My client Jack, fifty-four, asked me on Day Six of The Plan, "Is it just my imagination, or am I actually thinking more clearly than I have in years?" The answer was no; it wasn't his imagination at all. That's why we see people respond so quickly to their "trigger" foods, and why, once we get those foods out of their system and their diet, they see such rapid weight loss and such a dramatic decrease in symptomology. They look and feel better than they ever have. Douse the flames of inflammation and your body does what it was physiologically designed to do, which is achieve homeostasis.

The secret to unlocking the mystery of your unique chemistry is discovering the specific trigger foods that are setting off an inflammatory response. Identifying and eliminating those foods is the answer to losing weight, looking younger, and feeling your best. This is what The Plan is all about.

Marci, 56

Before The Plan, two to three bouts of terrible IBS every week were not uncommon for me. I could not pinpoint any foods in particular that were causing me problems, but I had learned what would relieve the symptoms: a hot bath and a glass of red wine. Many days my gut was in such distress I could barely make it to the end of the work day. Such pain! I thought I was eating a very healthy diet. I avoided most processed food, ate loads of vegetables and "healthy" whole grains, lean meat and fish, etc. In short, I thought I was doing everything "right" for my body. So why was I so miserable so much of the time?

The secret was in The Plan. I have had five (yes, just five) bouts of IBS symptoms over the past six months. This alone is amazing to me. No doctor could help me find relief, but The Plan has given me the tools to figure out what foods are compatible with my particular body and which ones are not. I have followed this way of eating ever since, and have been telling everyone who will sit still long enough to listen. I've also lost over ten pounds in the process, which is such a bonus!

I also introduced my twenty-two-year-old niece to The Plan last September. She had been diagnosed with a form of arthritis and was in such pain she had to sit down to go down the stairs. Her doctor wanted to put her on Humira, because the drug she was on, Enbrel, wasn't doing enough. I convinced her to give The Plan a try first. I just hated the idea of her being on such strong drugs at such a young age. My niece embraced The Plan with great dedication and enthusiasm. Today, she is off all her meds, and most days, symptom free.

Thanks, Lyn-Genet. You have changed my (and my niece's) life!

Trigger Foods

The most frustrating part of this is that you've probably been eating the very foods that are setting the whole inflammatory process ablaze in your body—*without knowing it*. I always say it's not the chocolate, or cheese, or wine, or even the cake and cookies that are making you overweight and sick. But it very well might be one of your go-to "healthy" foods that is.

Donna was in her early fifties and had very bad eczema. She was single and living in Los Angeles—just about the last place you'd want to have a visible skin condition. She had twelve to fifteen pounds she wanted to lose, but the eczema was what brought her to me. Eczema is an inflammatory condition, so I knew The Plan would help us uncover what was igniting it.

Donna followed the first three days of The Plan, which is a cleanse that incorporates only the most universally nonreactive foods. On the cleanse, people generally see a weight loss of anywhere from four to six pounds and a dramatic decrease in symptomology, and Donna was no exception. On Day Four she woke up five pounds lighter, but even more importantly, the eczema was gone. Completely. She was thrilled!

On Day Four, we plugged in one of her favorite snacks: raw almonds. What could be healthier, right? Well, about eight almonds and as many minutes later, Donna pulled her car off to the side of the road to text me: "My mouth is on FIRE!" Aha! From there it was no big surprise to see that she gained a pound and a half and all of her eczema returned by the next morning. Donna had been eating raw almonds instead of chocolate as a treat all along, never realizing that this "virtuous" snack was actually the source of her problems.

Chances are you've been eating one or more of your specific trigger foods for years, mistaking it for something healthy. But one of the fundamental and life-changing truths you'll learn from The Plan is this: **There is no such thing as healthy. There is only what works for *your* body.** Every person's chemistry is unique. What might set off an inflammatory response in your system and cause weight gain might be perfectly fine for someone else, and vice versa.

A lot of people call me the contrarian because I'm not touting the merits of "healthy" foods like salmon, or oatmeal, or asparagus. Don't get me wrong; I have nothing against these foods, if they work for you. But those are the key words right there: if they work for *you*. In the abstract, these foods might be considered healthy, or even superfoods, but for 85 percent of my clients over the age of thirty-five, they lead to weight gain and health issues (The Plan is geared toward people over the age of thirty-five or people with weakened digestion. As you'll read about shortly, unless a person has a chronic illness, foods will not generate the same amount of reactive response in those under thirty-five because we lose digestive enzymes as we age).

Common wisdom in the dieting world has taught us to believe

that some foods—usually the fun ones—are universally bad. So, if you're like most of the men and women I've worked with who are desperate to lose weight and improve their health, you start cutting those out. But they're usually not the problem. If they were, then you wouldn't be faced with the all-too-common mystery of eating "healthy" or drastically reducing calories and still gaining weight. How many times have you ordered plain grilled fish at a restaurant and thought, "Wow, I'm being so good," not knowing that every time you ate it you were gaining a pound? How many times have you opted for multigrain bread, not realizing that the corn or oats were causing your weight gain and health issues? At the same time, how often do you deprive yourself of the foods you love when in fact they might be better for you than Brussels sprouts or asparagus?

Believe me, I know what you're thinking. How can white bread be better for you than multigrain? Or potato chips better than bananas? It comes back to that fundamental truth that there is no such thing as universally healthy. We've all heard stories about people who lived well into their nineties eating steak, white bread, and butter. Clearly these foods are friendly for their chemistry. I wouldn't dare tell these people they have to switch to broccoli, it could kill them!

At the same time, I'll bet there's some "healthy" food that you've always secretly suspected wasn't working for you. Thirty-eight-year-old Ingrid frequently ordered steamed shrimp and vegetables from her local Chinese takeout place, until she discovered on The Plan that this "dietetic" option was behind her weight gain—and her achy knees to boot. Ted, forty-seven, lived off his signature "healthy" recipe of turkey meat loaf made with oats, peppers, and tomato sauce for years, until he realized that this combo would cause a three-pound weight gain. (Ted now refers to that retired recipe as his Weight Gain Meat Loaf Express.) Fifty-one-year-old Marguerite joked, "You mean I can finally stop eating those rice cakes that I swear make my stomach blow up like a balloon?"

Bridget, 39

Tomorrow I will be thirty-eight weeks pregnant with a surprise baby boy that I publicly credit to Lyn-Genet's Plan!

I was your garden-variety "unexplained" infertile. On paper, I was completely healthy: blood work never showed anything that explained the infertility. I had headaches, sporadic malaise, joint pain, and recurring bouts of anxiety and depression. I'd tried everything: skin tests for allergies, vegetarian living (for five years!), a gluten-free diet, even a raw diet. It got to the point that I was embarrassed to talk to friends about my latest nutritional experiments for fear of sounding like a total flake.

Our first daughter took thirty cycles to conceive. When she was eighteen months old, I began missing ovulation, having periods every ten days. After chasing our tails with my regular ob-gyn, we sought out a reproductive endocrinologist, who, again, diagnosed us as "unexplained infertility" and helped us conceive our second daughter with follicle-stimulating hormones and intrauterine insemination. But it wasn't until I was seven months pregnant that the really scary health events began. One day I looked up and couldn't read the television menu. I assumed it was common pregnancy-related vision fluctuations due to fluid retention. But it did not resolve with the pregnancy. When my youngest daughter was eight months old, we learned it was fluid retention on the occipital lobe of my brain.

The neurologist ruled out all scary and life-threatening causes (stroke, blood clots, tumors) and diagnosed me with migraines that had reached a transition stage. This meant that I was living with headaches every day for so long that I was no longer fully aware of them unless they flared as full-blown debilitating headaches or visual disturbance. I had two options: wean my baby girl and begin daily migraine suppressant medication, or try to see if I was allergic to anything in my diet. The neurologist was reluctant to ask me to begin doing anything that disrupted the development of my infant, but he also warned me that elimination diets were usually very tricky, often frustrating, and took a great deal of time to complete.

I was determined to fix this thing by eating. I ran out to our local market, bought everything organic in sight, and began eating "right." Two weeks later I was having some of the worst headaches of my adult life.

Enter Lyn-Genet. First I learned that the conventional media-backed "healthy" things I'd been eating while trying to obtain nutritional sainthood, such as dinners of salmon and Brussels sprouts with grapefruit juice spritzers, were actually some of the highest-reactionary foods I could ingest. That got my attention. Upon that revelation, Lyn had my total trust. We wasted no time and began my plan as soon as I could gather the necessary ingredients. (I live in rural Kentucky—but there was nothing on the list I couldn't procure within a few clicks.)

Within three days on The Plan, I began my first period. On Days Four and Five we identified sensitivities to tree nuts and buckwheat. But within seven days, we learned what my primary hidden reactive culprit was . . . *mustard*! And I was a mustard junkie. I rubbed it on meats, used it in salads, poured it on sandwiches. Who would ever have thought that spicy little grain would be so volatile for my health? But looking back, it made perfect sense. When I was a child, we would travel to the nearest big city to eat tempura-battered chicken fingers, which I would slather with honey-mustard dressing. Invariably, eleven-year-old me spent the car ride home with nausea and migraines.

Now, with a new vision for what I should include in and eliminate from my diet, weight began to fall off. I felt anxiety lift, life stressors eased, and the subtle details, like where I put my car keys, began to fall into focus. Forty days later, and seventeen pounds lighter, I found out I was pregnant.

I'll be honest: for me, pregnancy is a survival sport where this host lives on the demands of her growing boy (think Cheez-Its and Lucky Charms). So while I haven't stuck to The Plan through this gestation, I have continued to avoid the foods that I know my body cannot tolerate, because, quite simply, they've been proven to me to be of great harm. I look forward to getting back on The Plan and getting back to prebaby weight, but most importantly, being able to nurture and enjoy our family with a clear head and vigorous health.

The Accomplices

You didn't think inflammation did its dirty work all on its own, did you? It's clever, but not that clever. It's got a few evil sidekicks doing its bidding that make those extra pounds hang on for dear life.

The Madness of Metabolism

Jackie had been thin and fit her whole life. At five feet seven inches and 120 pounds, she could rock a pair of skinny jeans like nobody's business. She ate well and ran three to four times a week, and even though she worked full-time and had three little kids at home, she still had the energy of a teenager.

Until she turned forty-two.

Almost overnight, it seemed, everything changed. First came the dreaded muffin top. First a little one, then not so little. Those skinny jeans went from being her go-to sexy uniform to a denim torture device. So she did what she'd always done when she needed to drop a few pounds. She cut out the carbs, dumped her full-fat lattes for coffee with skim milk, and upped her cardio, but...nothing. Not a pound was budging. She started to experiment with a few of the popular diet programs, including going completely vegan and raw for two weeks, with nothing but a lot of gas and frustration to show for it. Like so many of my clients, Jackie felt completely at a dead end, wondering where her lifelong reliable metabolism had gone.

What we're dealing with here isn't metabolism. It's aging as an inflammatory process. That's right: aging itself is an inflammatory process. When our bodies stop burning certain foods as a calorie in/calorie out, various systems start to slow down, including hormonal, digestive, cognitive, immune, etc. That's why our health degenerates as we get older. Inflammation and its effects are cumulative over time, and our response to food changes as our inflammatory state increases.

At the age of twenty-five, most of us hit what I call our first inflammatory speed bump. A hundred calories of green beans will now process in our body like 150 calories, and perhaps we notice that we start to gain weight and have problems with digestion. So we start to exercise more or eat a little healthier, and we're able to moderate our weight that way. That's why it's so easy to lose weight in our twenties; cut out a cookie a day and the weight slides right off.

Then, at age thirty-five, that same 100-calorie food acts like 700 calories if it's reactive for you. This is when we start to experience more dramatic health issues. The gas that we suffered from in our twenties can become chronic constipation, celiac disease, or IBS in our thirties. Ages forty-two and fifty are when we really see the major shift, with a 100-calorie food that you're reactive to registering in your body as 3,500 to 7,000 calories. Now those digestive issues can become a risk for colon cancer. And as we know, the foods you're reactive to are usually the ones you least suspect—thus, you can mysteriously gain two pounds after eating a small bowl of Greek yogurt. Identifying this "mysterious" weight gain is the most vital key to your health.

When I first developed The Plan, my client base was thirty-five to forty-five years old, and I'd see usually three to four foods show up as reactive for them. As the clients' ages increased beyond forty-two, however, I'd see them react to many more, because their bodies were already in a state of low-grade, chronic inflammation from years of eating "healthy" foods. If you keep eating foods that you don't know are reactive for you at a younger age, you'll be more prone to making even more foods reactive later on. Let's say that at twenty-five, you're slightly reactive to tomato sauce and high-gluten bread. But you don't know it, so you eat pizza three nights a week for years. Then you're forty-five, and because you've created an inflammatory state in your body to begin with, suddenly eggplant, fish, sweet potatoes, and eggs are also now food sensitivities for you.

The longer you take to identify your reactive foods, the more extreme the state of chronic, low-grade inflammation becomes, causing premature aging, weight gain, and disease. The bad news is that inflammation can have a domino effect, so what was PMS now becomes hormonal disorders. Frequent headaches turn into chronic migraines and depression. As the effects increase, your weight increases right along with them.

The good news is that when you reduce or reverse the inflammatory state by eliminating your reactive foods, you can radically and quickly reverse illness, weight gain—and even the aging process itself.

The Mother of All Hormone Regulators

The thyroid is a major player when it comes to hormonal health, since it stimulates and synchronizes all cellular functions—primarily metabolism.

I would say about 80 percent of my female clients in their forties and 10 percent of my male clients are thyroid dysfunctional. Of those percentages, more than half of them don't even know it. The standard thyroid-stimulating hormone (TSH) test used by doctors misses a lot of cases of hypothyroidism because it's just looking at a specific number. If your TSH is above 3.0, you have hypothyroidism; if it isn't, you don't. But people aren't just their numbers, and thousands are going undiagnosed. By the time the lab numbers show a problem, you already need medication and you've been suffering for years. (FYI, the TRH, free T3, reverse T3, anti-TPO, antithyroglobulin, and free T4 tests are much better indicators. Doctors will do them if you ask, but you have to push for it.) Regardless of what markers register on tests, whenever the thyroid isn't operating at optimal levels, you can be sure that weight gain and low energy levels won't be far behind.

Estrogen domianance has a lot to do with hampering the thyroid. We often see hormonal imbalances during times of dramatic hormonal shift, like postpartum and in perimenopause, and when estrogen levels are higher than progesterone, it lowers the levels of free thyroid hormone in the body. Hormonal birth control pills (especially ones that limit monthly cycles), hormonal replacement therapy, and selective serotonin reuptake inhibitors (SSRIs) are definitely major contributing factors, as well as the onslaught of xenoestrogens we're exposed to on a daily basis in this country. They're in everything from pesticides to plastic bottles to shampoo and cosmetics. The lavender and tea tree oil in your skin care products are strong phytoestrogens—so much so that many endocrinologists are recommending you avoid these ingredients completely.

And don't even get me started on soy, which is a strong phytoestrogen. Food companies are adding soy to everything they can think of because it's an inexpensive way to boost protein, and consumers have bought into the hype of soy as a superfood. But excess soy has a huge effect on our hormonal balance—so much so that studies show that baby girls who are fed soy via formula are developing breast buds by the age of two. If that doesn't tell us that something's gone awry, I don't know what does. Will soy affect men as well? You bet it will!

Chronic low-grade inflammation, as you already know, is the basis for every disease. So certainly if your mother has thyroid dysfunction, or went through early menopause, inflammation is likely to kick-start thyroid issues for you. Or maybe you started birth control at sixteen, or Prozac at twenty-five, or are vegan and eat tons of soy products. All along, you're also unknowingly eating your reactive foods, priming the inflammatory state that will eventually trigger the latent thyroid problem. And because the thyroid is responsible for so many metabolic functions, your body is then set off on a roller coaster of health and weight issues.

Thankfully, it's very easy to determine whether your thyroid isn't operating as it should (I'll walk you through this in Part Two), and there are lots of things you can do to quickly boost its function. You want to find out and address this early so you can reverse a thyroid issue nutritionally, before it progresses to full-blown hypothyroidism.

A lot of people get freaked out at the idea of having a dysfunctional thyroid, but truthfully, it's not a big deal once you're aware of it. It's nothing more to worry about than having curly hair or straight hair. It's just how your body is wired, and I'll show you in a holistic way how to manipulate the variables in your favor.

The Sneaky Saboteur: Sodium

Sodium is needed by the body for daily function, but too much can greatly exacerbate an inflammatory response. Think of it like putting a match to the fuse on a stick of dynamite. Excess sodium in the body takes a mildly reactive food and turns it into a wildly reactive one.

Sodium is hidden in everything from breakfast cereals to salad dressing. We would expect to find it in foods like frozen meals and deli meats, but sodium is everywhere! Restaurant food is notoriously high in hidden salt. You can easily have three days' worth of sodium in one dinner out without knowing it. Even that plain poached chicken breast that seems so virtuous is likely cooked in chicken broth that's loaded with sodium and MSG.

In 2012, the Centers for Disease Control and Prevention released its list of the foods that are the highest source of sodium in the US diet, and the top of that list isn't the obvious guess of bacon or salty snack foods—it's bread. Next on the list of offenders are cold cuts and cured meats, then pizza, poultry, soups, sandwiches, cheese, pasta dishes, meat dishes, and salty snacks. With these being the staples of the American diet, it's no wonder so many people are way above the American Heart Association's current recommended daily amount of 1,500 milligrams.

On The Plan, we're going to easily get the excess sodium out of your diet. I promise, you won't miss it. The three-day initial cleanse will reset your palate so you're more attuned to the wonderful flavors in all different kinds of foods. Plus, as an added bonus, studies have shown that when you decrease your sodium intake, you curb sugar cravings. That's not to say that there's anything wrong with having sugar. I just don't want sugar to be the boss of you!

Water Shortage

I will be like the mother you never wanted when it comes to water. For weight loss, it is *essential* to drink approximately half your body weight in ounces. If you have even one glass less than your daily allotment, you'll see it show up on the scale. For every sixteen ounces less than your body needs, it will hold on to half a pound. I've seen this happen to my clients, again and again. If you're gaining half a pound, let's at least have it be from a decadent dessert—not a lack of water.

Water is needed for every metabolic and cellular function in your body. When you don't drink enough, your body has to extract water from your food and hold on to a reservoir in your cells to keep you alive. That takes energy, and your body only has so much energy. When you don't drink enough water, you're essentially telling your body, "Don't repair my heart, my liver, my lungs. Instead, I need you to use your energy to extract water from all the food I'm eating and hold on to it in my tissues." When you do drink enough, the body can let go of the extra water it's been holding on to, and the numbers on the scale go down. Feeling tired all the time? Try increasing your water and see how much more energy you have once you've taken away an extra "task" from the body and freed up your energy reserves.

When you don't drink enough water, you also increase an inflammatory response. I had a client who tested mahimahi and gained .2 pounds, signaling slight reactivity. (Anything less than a half-pound daily weight loss on The Plan signals reactivity.) But she loved fish, so we tested it again the next week. Everything else was the same that day as the prior week, minus four glasses of water. The result: a gain of three pounds, going from mildly reactive to wildly reactive in negative four glasses. Of course, when we see an exponential response to a low-calorie health food, we always see a health issue crop up, so this poor woman was constipated for three days!

Increase your water intake and the results can be dramatic. Estelle, sixty-one, was drinking only two glasses of water a day when she came to me weighing 163, wanting to lose twenty pounds. I told her to wait a week to start on The Plan, and in the meantime, simply increase her water intake to eighty ounces per day. Seven days later, without any other dietary changes whatsoever, she weighed 157 pounds. Six pounds disappeared just from drinking enough water. How's that for a little hydration motivation?

With all these things going wrong, it's no wonder so many people feel frustrated, upset, and angry. But it's time to change all that. It's time to finally unlock the mystery and take back control of your weight and health, with real information and real results.

Jayne, 50

2010 was not a healthy year for me; getting older is not an easy task sometimes.

I was diagnosed with an autoimmune disease (relapsing polychondritis, or RP) and polycystic ovarian syndrome a few years ago. RP is an inflammatory disease that, among other things, attacks the cartilage and cartilage-like organs in your body (joints, nose, ears, eyes, heart, lungs—real fun stuff). The prognosis is not good, and I was looking for anything I could do to slow down the progression. I took a total of seventeen pills every day.

I read about Lyn-Genet's anti-inflammatory program and it made a lot of sense to me. I had to try something to gain control over health issues that threatened to make my future not so bright. I also liked the idea that while there are general guidelines to The Plan, it has to be tailored to each person's personal reactions to food. No two people are the same.

I am not overweight, but I just wasn't comfortable with the increasing weight gain over the past several years. I have eaten healthy and organic for the last ten years but have not been able to lose any weight, even with Pilates, spinning, and working out at the gym regularly each week. I have had to take prednisone over the course of the last year for the RP, and that is an automatic ten-pound weight gain each course. If one more person said to me, "Oh, you look fine for your age. You're supposed to gain weight as you get older," I was going to throttle them. I just turned fifty—it isn't a death sentence!

Two and a half months into The Plan, I have lost over fifteen pounds, I feel great, and my skin looks fabulous (take that, fifty!). The doctors have taken me off the 2,500 milligrams of Metformin that I took on a daily basis for the PCOS. My RP has stayed the same, but I am no worse—and that is something! I believe that by following The Plan, I can do something organically to help my body fight this autoimmune disease. I am no longer a bystander but an active participant in my treatment.

CHAPTER TWO

The Plan to Right What's Going Wrong

The Plan isn't a diet. It's a complete change of mind-set. What you learn here in these twenty days will radically change the way you look at diets, your daily weight, and food.

I'll admit it: even though I read all the research and studies, I don't believe anything is true unless I've tested it on my own. I didn't set out to prove that the so-called healthy foods that are the lore and legend of nutrition programs everywhere were behind unexplained weight gain and health issues. Believe me, I didn't *want* foods like eggs and oatmeal to be reactive. I love eggs and oatmeal! But as I kept observing and recording what I was seeing, the results were showing up again and again, and I eventually connected the dots.

The seeds of what later became The Plan were planted when I was in my teens. I suffered from migraines almost daily, and at the age of fourteen I decided to take charge. I became a vegetarian and started practicing yoga, and turned myself from a low-energy, slightly depressed teen into someone who felt great all the time.

Ever since, I've immersed myself in the study of holistic nutrition, along with homeopathy, Eastern medicine, and herbology. I moved from my hometown of New York City to San Francisco, where I started working as a nutritionist, specializing in using diet and herbs to help with systemic yeast, hormones, and immunity response. The West Coast was a great place to get exposed to many different healthy food theories and diets, and I tried them all. With each one I tried, I thought I'd find what the "right" way to eat was. I slowly started to realize that all these diets and theories exist because they are "right" and work for a certain population, but that no one way of eating is the right fit for everyone.

Living in San Francisco awoke in me a love of seasonal and local produce, fantastic breads, and great wines. The colors, flavors, and vibrancy of the food really struck a chord. And so when I moved back home to New York, I pursued this passion, working as a manager and sommelier at two of New York City's hottest restaurants. Being surrounded by wonderful food and wine there, as well, proved my hunch that you can eat well and care for yourself at the same time.

After a few years, I left the restaurant business to explore new paths. I opened a small yoga studio downtown, working with women on pre- and postnatal health, and later ran a physical therapy center for rehabilitation. When people came to me in pain, I of course always made nutritional suggestions. So many people were asking for my nutritional advice that I eventually opened a small private practice. As that grew, and as I identified a deep personal need to help my home community, I opened a holistic health center in Harlem serving hundreds of people each week.

Working intensely with the diverse population of Harlem, I started noticing that when I suggested to my clients many of the usual healthy foods to lose weight, their weight actually went up rather than down. If we're not changing the caloric value for the day as a whole, there's no reason someone should gain a full pound or two from a 200-calorie healthy food, and so I started to investigate.

I communicated with my clients daily, monitoring their weight and health issues. I noticed repeatedly that when they would put on half a pound or more, a health or emotional issue would crop up as well. The symptoms would vary from person to person, ranging from minor aches and pains, to feeling down, to full-blown migraines, but there was a notable correlation between a weight bump and these reactions. When there was a reaction, I'd help them find the clues: when did the bloating, the depressed feeling, or the headache start? What did they eat that might have triggered it?

I treated every client as an individual in terms of potentially reactive food choices, but there were common themes that were hard to ignore. Eighty-five percent of them were gaining weight when they ate salmon or black beans—and that just seemed too much of a coincidence. I started compiling lists about the odds of foods causing a weight bump, and sure enough, I saw consistent information.

I'd been studying all the research on inflammation, so I knew that inflammation happens instantaneously. (Think about it: you cut yourself and the area immediately becomes red and inflamed; that's the healing inflammatory process at work.) Hmm...okay, so I knew inflammation was the basis of all disease, and that it had been linked to weight gain. The Plan has a pretty consistent caloric content each day, so if my clients one day plugged in a healthy food like tomato sauce and almost immediately saw a health condition like arthritis flare up and an overnight gain of two pounds, that had to be an inflammatory response, right? All the information and research was out there connecting inflammation to weight gain, but no one was putting the pieces together and identifying foods as the trigger.

I couldn't understand why no one was really addressing this in the medical or nutritional community, so I started to really home in on my own research and testing. I continued to communicate with my clients daily—sometimes hourly—closely monitoring their new food variables and corresponding health/weight response. I listened closely to everything they were telling me in order to identify the patterns and triggers. Pretty soon I realized that the reason more people weren't studying this was because, frankly, it took a lot of work in the beginning to develop a testing protocol! But after all my research and study and seeing the results with my own eyes, I knew I'd found the answer I'd been looking for.

I had probably worked with over three hundred clients by the time the basics of The Plan took shape. Today my staff of naturo-pathic doctors and nutritionists and I work with more than two thousand clients a year from all over the world. No matter where they're from, or how different their circumstances, again and again I have witnessed this anti-inflammatory practice changing people's lives.

Laura, 44

Since I was about fifteen years old, nothing has annoyed me more than being told that if I just exercised more and ate a little less I would lose weight and have more energy. Obvious, but completely unhelpful.

I was diagnosed with fibromyalgia, Epstein-Barr, and chronic fatigue in my early twenties. At times, just getting out of bed and showering were miraculous feats of athleticism. Gosh, even sleeping could be exhausting. But yes, you are probably right that I would feel much better if I would just stop being so lazy and go out and run a 5K. Silly me.

I was always the big girl. Usually the largest of all my friends, with a wardrobe full of practical clothes that fit rather than the cute and sassy clothes I really wanted to wear.

If there was a weight loss diet out there that promised to give me more energy and caused the weight to fall off—sign me up! I haven't stopped experimenting to find a way to eat that would make me feel better since I was fifteen. I've done the four food groups, and protein diets, and Weight Watchers, and raw food, and brown rice diets, and candida diets, and allergy and elimination diets. On some of them I temporarily dropped a few pounds, but none of them ever really eased the fatigue or pain. It felt like a vicious cycle of health and weight struggles because I was obviously just too lazy to do what it took to have energy and be pain free.

Until now.

After spending the last three months playing detective with this amazing process developed by Lyn-Genet that lets you easily pinpoint the foods that create chronic inflammation in your system, I am thirty-five pounds lighter, five sizes smaller...and pain free. I eat cheese, dark chocolate, and—wait for it—potato chips.

Take that!

It didn't require exercising more or eating less. In fact, I exercise less and eat more. It required understanding my own chemistry and getting to the bottom of what foods stress my system and create inflammation (which showed up for me as depression, pain, fatigue, and extra weight). And mine is only one of thousands of stories of people who have changed their health and their life with this incredible technique.

The Anti-Diet

If you're looking for another "Tell me what to eat and I'll eat it" program, you're going to be disappointed. Oh, if only it were as easy as my saying, "Here's a list of reactive foods. Don't eat them and you'll lose weight." Sure, I could do that, but *wow*, would your life be boring—and you'd probably be right back looking for the next diet in six months.

This is actually the anti-diet. I don't want to teach you to eat like me or like any of my clients who have lost weight. I want to teach you to eat like *you*, according to what works for *your* individual body. The main reason standard diet plans don't work is that they're the exact opposite of personalized. They're simply an average of what doctors or dietitians have found. I'll give you an example. Everyone loses weight on chicken. Everyone loses weight on rice. So chicken and rice get put onto the "good foods" list. But when we combine chicken and rice in one meal, 80 percent of my clients have an inflammatory response. If I were a diet maven, I'd simply say, "Don't eat chicken and rice." But how do I know whether you're in the 80 percent or the 20 percent? If it's a combination that works fine for you, why shouldn't you have it?

Just because a food is reactive for 80 percent of my clients doesn't mean it's going to be reactive for you. I love it when people turn out to be in the 20 percent! Plus, once you reverse the inflammation in your body, you'll be able to enjoy in moderation foods that you might be reactive to, because you've reduced that inflammatory pathway.

Another big reason diets don't work is because no one likes to be told what to do. If I were to tell you not to eat pizza because it would make you gain weight, you'd probably hate me for it. You might even avoid pizza for a while, but then the craving would return and you'd climb right back on the unhealthy roller coaster of giving in to cravings, weight gain, guilt, deprivation…and on it would go. But if I teach you how to test pizza, you have in your hands the proof of how this food reacts for you, and then you're the one who gets to choose.

You don't ever have to give up on a food you love, even if it's reactive for you. There's always a way! I once worked with a great woman named Dina, then forty-six, who had debilitating arthritic pain. By Day Nine of The Plan her arthritis was in complete remission and she was down six pounds, enjoying 2,200 calories a day. Then the confession came out: "Lyn," she said, "I looooove pizza. Please don't tell me I need to stop eating pizza to keep losing weight!" I heard her loud and clear, so I said we should test her on the components of pizza. We tested her on the bread: she lost half a pound. We tested her on cheese: another half pound. I waited to test her on tomato sauce because I know tomato sauce is the devil, and sure enough, when she tested it, Dina went up two pounds and all of her arthritic pain returned for forty-eight hours. Dina was devastated, thinking this meant no more pizza, ever. I told her to hang on and suggested an alternative of white pizza. She was thrilled beyond belief! Today she's at her goal weight, free of pain, loving her white pizza.

On The Plan, we let your tastes and your body's reactions dictate what to test. As one of my clients said, "I love The Plan—especially because it's all about *me*!"

It's About Chemistry, Not Calories

Weight loss isn't about portion size.

It's not about calories.

It's all about chemistry.

Most people who come to me ask the usual questions about a diet, like how many calories or carbs or fat grams they can have per day. But I tell them repeatedly that we don't know anything until they go through The Plan and test. Ultimately, it doesn't matter how many calories you're eating for weight loss, as long as you're eating foods that burn clean *for you* (ie, are nonreactive). Reactive calories will put on weight, but what I call clean calories won't.

We don't know what the correct caloric intake is for most people, but it's probably more than you're eating. People are constantly under-eating and not getting enough calories to fuel their bodies properly. Using the standard protocol for my height and weight, I should be eating 1,100 calories a day. But I eat 2,000 or more calories a day. My weight stays steady and I feel healthy and energized, because I'm eating the foods that work for my body. But if I have even one egg (one of my highly reactive foods), my allergies will kick up, I'll look six months pregnant, and I'll put on a pound. Seventy calories from one egg, and look what happens. And I used to *love* eggs! They worked just great for me up until the age of thirty-five. Not anymore, though. It's a no-brainer. It's amazing how your desires change once you discover the foods that are making you put on weight and feel unwell.

Billie, fifty-three, had finished her Plan a month before her birthday rolled around. Billie notoriously loved cupcakes and was worried about what would happen on her birthday because she knew everyone would bring her favorite treat. I told her to go ahead and enjoy herself—we're meant to have fun! The next morning, Billie emailed me and said she was scared to step on the scale because she'd eaten four or five large cupcakes. I tough-mothered her into it, because as you'll learn very shortly, the scale isn't the enemy. Would you believe she didn't gain a single pound? Again: chemistry, not calories. Her body did just fine with cake because she had been working The Plan in her everyday life surrounding the cupcake day, and she wasn't reactive to any of the ingredients. If you eat according to your Plan, you strengthen your digestive system; this allows you to have a day completely off the charts. Your body will process the foods with minimal reaction, and then you can get right back on your Plan!

I'm here to help you figure out your own body's chemistry so you can know definitively which are your "friendly" foods and which ones are "reactive" for you. I want to change the methodology of thinking that says you can't have foods you enjoy. You can have any food you want and lose weight, if that food works for you and you find the right balance. The day a client tells me (and soon this will be you) that he or she knows calories mean nothing is the day I know that client *owns* his or her Plan.

So many of us who are conscious eaters have been slowly cutting out joyful foods and never think of reintroducing them. It's funny how many Italian clients I've had who have told me they'd forgotten how good olive oil is. But enjoyment of food really is a key element of the "chemistry, not calories" equation. There's a reason why Billie ate five cupcakes on her birthday and didn't gain an ounce. When you're out with friends and family, having fun and laughing, foods don't process the same as when you're sitting at home feeling depressed, counting your bites and worrying about calories. Having fun emotionally allows you to have some fun gastronomically. I've seen this play out so many times on The Plan. Savoring and living joyously is one of the best ways to alchemize your body's chemistry in your favor.

Your Daily Weight Is Nothing More Than Data

The very thing you've come to hate—the scale—is actually your best friend. It's a key tool for determining how your body responds to food. You just need to learn to interpret what the numbers are telling you.

Your weight each day is nothing more than data. There's no magic to it. I know, right now the ups and downs of your weight feel like a frustrating mystery. But there's *always* an explanation, every single day, for why your weight is what it is, and knowing what that explanation is puts you back in control.

A pound weight gain is not personal, and we need to stop taking it that way. It's simply your body's response to one or several foods that don't work for you. That's all. I want you to think of the next twenty days as a controlled science experiment. We're going to objectively gather data that will help you know how and what to eat for the rest of your life. It's hard, I know, because a gain in weight hits all the emotional buttons. But I'm not going to let you get hung up on the number on the scale. In the past, maybe if you weighed yourself and you'd gained a pound, you'd get demoralized—it might even ruin your entire day. But on The Plan, it's just data. And like a scientist, you have to distance yourself from the data.

Let's say that yesterday, you tested mozzarella, and today you're up half a pound. You could get upset by that, and of course it's hard when you see the scale register a gain or stabilization. But all that number tells us is valuable information about what mozzarella does for your body. Does that mean you can't ever have mozzarella? Of course not. As I said, I don't ever want you to give up on foods that you love. Sure, you can choose not to eat mozzarella, or you can find ten other cheeses that don't make you gain, or plug mozzarella in on a day after you've lost half a pound. You'll learn how to do all of this in the days to come.

If you test a food and it's friendly for you, fantastic. If it's reactive, you'll know that, too, and be able to make informed choices about how to work it into your life. From now on, whether it's mozzarella, pizza, cupcakes, eggs, or anything else, you're in the driver's seat.

How The Plan Works

By now you're probably wondering how you're going to lose all that weight I promised you would. It's simple, actually. We systematically test foods from the least reactive on up. While about 30 percent of your days might show a reactive response and weight bump (remember, it's all just data), the other 70 percent will be amazing days for you as you add to your list of "friendly" foods. Find forty to fifty foods that work for you and you'll be at your goal weight. When we eliminate the reactive foods and create delicious meals with our friendly ones, the weight flies off faster than we ever thought possible.

The first three days are Phase One of The Plan. You'll do an easy detox cleanse that incorporates the least reactive foods, to set a base line. You'll still be eating three full meals and a snack each day, consuming 2,200 to 2,600 calories (for women) or 2,800 to 3,400 calories (for men), so you won't be at all hungry.

Day Four begins Phase Two of The Plan. We'll begin systematically testing foods from the least reactive to the most reactive, to determine which are friendly for you. We insert one new item approximately every other day, be it a food or a dish at a restaurant you love. I will give you general guidelines for what to test, and throughout will encourage you to test the foods (and drinks) that matter most to you. If you love steak, we'll test that. Cheese? Absolutely. Pancakes? Sure thing. Scotch? Not a problem. You can test anything that is part of your life. Like I said, this isn't my Plan—it's your Plan. We're going to help you learn to eat like *you*.

All the way through, you'll learn how to interpret your body's signals, because they will tell us everything we need to know. You'll know precisely why you've gained, lost, or stabilized, how to assess your body's clues to determine whether a new variable is friendly or reactive for you, and if you do have a reactive response, exactly what to do to reverse that quickly and get right back on track.

Phase Three, the final stage of The Plan, is where you'll learn everything you need to know to test on your own. I'll teach you the basics of creating balanced daily menus so that you can easily test any new food or restaurant menu going forward and get accurate results.

By the time we're done, you're going to know for certain which foods do and do not work for your body. You're going to discover and eliminate, once and for all, the ones that are triggering the inflammatory response responsible for your weight gain and health issues. You'll build your arsenal of friendly foods you can joyfully choose from whenever you need to reliably lose weight, and create a personalized eating plan you can use to keep your body slim, healthy, and energized—for the rest of your life.

John, 47

Between a hectic work schedule and the desire to be a good dad and husband, I don't have the time for nor interest in dieting—but I do care a lot about my health. I'm also an amateur triathlete, so fitness and energy levels matter a lot. The Plan doesn't tell me how to diet; it helps me figure out the best foods to eat to promote a healthy, energetic state of being. The Plan's approach is strictly tailored to me, both in terms of evaluating what foods make my body happy and providing the encouragement and nutritional science behind why my body acts the way it does. The Plan is so easy to work with, but best of all, I can look and feel better!

Part Two

THE PLAN FOR WEIGHT LOSS AND HEALTH

CHAPTER THREE

Prepping for The Plan

Welcome to your Plan!

In just twenty days from now, you'll be well on your way to reaching your goals of eating healthier, feeling refreshed and energized, and—of course—losing weight. But before we dive in, let's run through the short list of things you need to know and supplies you'll want to have on hand to set you up for maximum success.

What You'll Need

You don't need much to get started on The Plan. There are no special foods or shakes to buy, no counter scale needed to weigh your food. The goal is to make your enjoyment of food greater, not fill your cabinets and body with fake food or burden you with measuring and counting.

Here's the short list of basic supplies you'll need:

- **A digital bathroom scale.** Remember, the scale is your new best friend. You'll want to find a digital scale that registers weight by tenths of a pound (some older models round up or down to the nearest half pound). I recommend the EatSmart scale, which is available online and relatively inexpensive.

- **A basal body temperature thermometer.** This will be the key tool for determining your thyroid function. You can find a digital thermometer at your local drugstore (many have them displayed in the family planning section, as they are used for determining ovulation cycles).

- **Basic cooking utensils.** You're going to be doing some easy cooking at home, so you want to make sure your kitchen is ready to go. You don't need to go crazy here. A large sauté pan or wok, a Dutch oven, a roasting pan or large baking dish, and basic utensils will suffice. In the summertime or in year-round warm climates, break out the grill if you have one.

- **A notebook or journal.** This will become your Plan Journal for the twenty days, where you'll record all your stats, body responses, and so on. It's important to keep a record of the data you collect, since it will become the blueprint for your new way of life. You can also download a weight loss sheet at www.lyngenet.com.

Julie, 53

I've lost more than twenty-four pounds on The Plan after trying for twenty years to lose weight. I followed every weight loss program you can imagine. I would lose five or so pounds and then it would all stop. Everyone always asked me the same question, skeptically: "Are you sure you are following the program?" I would leave in tears because I *was* following the programs!

Then by a miracle I found an article about Lyn in a magazine. I called her right away and within a few months I was on The Plan. All those years I had been eating great diet foods like salmon and green beans, thinking I was doing what was right. Now I know that I am reactive to those foods—and many others. The most important thing that I learned is that there are a lot of foods that actually are friendly foods for me…good regular food! I *don't* diet anymore. I am truly free of that word. I'm really living now! I live and love The Plan. My blood work shows so much improvement, my blood pressure is the lowest it's been in my life, my psoriasis is gone, the IBS I suffered all of my adult life is gone. The Plan has truly helped me change my life.

Supplements

Let me say this right up front: I'm not big on supplements. People load up on every vitamin, mineral, enzyme, and more under the sun, and truthfully, it's a little ridiculous. You shouldn't need all of that if you're eating well. On The Plan, I assure you you're going to get all the nutrients you need.

Having said that, we may use a few specific supplements during the initial stages of The Plan to get the body into its optimal non-inflammatory state (or as needed throughout in short doses). I don't believe in taking any kind of supplement for the long term. The goal is to take whatever you need when you need it, let it do its job, then stop to allow your body to self-regulate. You hear all the time about supplements that are supposedly great, and then years later hear that they've been proven ineffective—or even that there's a health risk involved. For instance, a study funded by the National Cancer Institute and published in 2011 in the *Journal of the American Medical Association* revealed that vitamin E, once touted as an important antioxidant, showed a 17 percent increased risk for men of developing prostate cancer. Another study published in the same year in the *Archives of Internal Medicine* showed that multivitamins gradually contribute to higher mortality rates in women, rather than making us healthier as they are purported to do. Additionally, so many people eat foods that are already fortified with supplements, thus increasing their chance of going over the safety limits of vitamins like B3 and B6.

As a general rule, it's better to give your body a break periodically from any kind of supplement or vitamin to allow it to reset itself. I personally like to cycle in and out of different nutritional or herbal remedies as my body needs them. If I'm feeling under the weather, I'll take zinc for a day. For sinus problems, I'll use a short dosage of MSM (more on that below). During periods where I know I will be under stress for a big work project, I'll take SAM-e. (SAM-e is a naturally occurring substance in the body that creates chemicals to help the body with stress, anxiety, depression, chronic pain, and liver dysfunction. It is also used for Alzheimer's, dementia, chronic fatigue syndrome and Parkinson's disease.)

For the purposes of beginning The Plan, I recommend the following:

- **Liver detoxifier (or dandelion tea).** The liver is responsible for over five hundred functions, including metabolism and hormonal control. We see big changes right away on The Plan when people start supporting their liver health, especially during the initial three-day detox. You can either drink one cup of dandelion tea, which is known for its liver-healing properties, or take a detox supplement, both of which are available at most natural food stores. (If you are on prescription medications, you may want to consider the detox supplement; herbs are wonderful, but they take longer to have an effect.) I've found NOW Liver Detoxifier & Regenerator or milk thistle to be the most effective liver support supplements. The recommended dosage is three capsules daily. If you want to continue to take the liver cleanser on a regular basis after the twenty days (I do), that's fine. We're exposed to so many environmental toxins and pesticides that the liver can always use a little extra love. Just take a week or two off every two months or so to allow the body to reset.

- **MSM.** Ah, the savior for people with allergies! MSM (methylsulfonylmethane) is a natural form of sulfur that can reset the entire histamine response in your body (which, in turn, reduces your response to foods). MSM strengthens mucosa and makes it resistant to external allergens. It's amazing how often I see people who are severely overweight who also suffer from allergies. What's the correlation? You guessed it: inflammation. If you have a history of food allergies or asthma, you'll want to take anywhere from 3,000 to 6,000 milligrams for six weeks. Personally, MSM has changed my life. I suffered from allergies, which would trigger sinus infections and then migraines. I took MSM for the recommended six-week course, and it knocked out those sinus infections for five years. When they started to reappear, I took one dose and I was good for another year. I highly recommend trying MSM for allergies or sinus issues so we can reverse that inflammation at the outset. The more inflammatory your state when you enter your Plan, the more sensitive you will be to your reactive foods. Decreasing your histamine response at the beginning will mean more weight loss and better health.

- **Probiotics.** One of the hallmarks of a reactive response is constipation. Clients constantly ask what they can do to alleviate it, and the answer is to take probiotics when it happens, to rebalance the digestive system. Constipation may not be an issue for you, but I like to have clients get probiotics in advance so they have them in hand, just in case. Probiotics are also very effective for balancing a yeast overgrowth, which we'll talk about shortly. In addition, taking a probiotic as soon as you notice gas or bloating will ease digestion and lessen weight gain from reactive food. You'll want to get one that has 30 to 50 billion live cultures in it. Some on the market go up to 200 billion, but that's not necessary. We have found ReNew Life, which you can find at any health food store, to be the most effective brand overall.

Testing Your Thyroid

Thyroid dysfunction can show up in many different ways. Most people with an underactive thyroid will, however, display some if not all of these symptoms:

- Inability to lose weight
- Fatigue
- Depression
- Feeling cold
- Digestive problems
- Low sex drive
- Hormonal imbalance
- Skin conditions

Before you begin your Plan, we'll want to get a reading on your thyroid so we know whether it's functioning up to par. It's actually very easy to test yourself for an underactive thyroid—no blood test needed.

For three days before beginning The Plan, keep your digital thermometer by your bed at night. When you wake up in the morning, place the thermometer in your armpit and hold it there for two to three minutes, to get a read on your basal body temperature (BBT). Keep still; moving around will raise your body temperature and throw off the reading.

A consistent temperature of 97 degrees Fahrenheit or lower is indicative of an underactive thyroid. I've found repeatedly that when temperatures are below that level, it's harder to lose weight, and all the systems are affected in a negative way. Some clients are surprised to see their body temperatures show up in the low range; they never even considered that their thyroid was behind a range of "mystery" problems they've been living with. But then again, many others aren't surprised at all. I can't tell you how many times I've heard, "That explains *so* much!"

I'd say about 80 percent of women in their forties I work with and about 10 percent of the men at that age have thyroid issues. That's a high statistic, but the good news is that when you identify the dysfunction before it gets to full-blown hypothyroidism, it's easily reversible.

Here is the simple protocol for boosting thyroid function:

- **Kelp**. Kelp is high in iodine, which is terrific for boosting thyroid function. Often doctors and nutritionists say not to take kelp supplements because seaweed attracts toxins to it. Indeed, if you take kelp that comes from polluted waters, you'll basically be poisoning yourself, so you want to choose your brand wisely. We recommend Norwegian kelp, which is the cleanest source; my preferred brand is NOW Foods. If your BBT is below 96 take 150–250 micrograms each morning with your breakfast until we start to see your BBT consistently at or above 97 degrees and/or your symptoms abate. Some people will stabilize at 96.5, but if you're losing weight at a normal pace and feeling good, that's absolutely fine. Everyone's base line is different; what matters most is what feels optimal for your body.

- **Maine Coast Sea Seasonings**. Some of my favorite seasonings for thyroid health are Maine Coast Sea Seasonings, another excellent source of iodine. I like this brand in particular because Maine Coast regularly tests their products for toxins. Maine Coast Sea Seasonings' seaweed is very flavorful. It comes in a shaker and is a great alternative to salt. For many of my clients, Maine Coast Sea Seasonings become a favorite way to spice up all kinds of dishes.

- **B12 supplements**. Liquid B12 is known for helping with energy levels, detoxing the liver, and improving thyroid function. However, taken for too long, it can overload your adrenal system, creating bodily stress that leads to weight gain. So again, we're talking about a contained course here until your thyroid function improves. I recommend NOW B12 Complex.

- **Avoid goitrogenic foods (until we test them)**. Goitrogens are compounds found in certain foods that have been shown to interfere with thyroid function by blocking the enzymes, which helps produce thyroid hormones. Many people who have thyroid disease are able to eat some foods on the goitrogen list with no ill effects whatsoever, but eating raw goitrogenic foods is generally more problematic. (Note that cooking often deactivates goitrogens, especially broccoli and kale.)

The most common goitrogenic foods are:

Broccoli
Broccoli rabe
Brussels sprouts
Cabbage
Cauliflower
Collards
Horseradish
Kale
Mustard
Rutabaga
Turnips
Millet
Peaches
Peanuts
Pine nuts
Radishes
Raspberries
Soybean and soy products, including tofu
Spinach
Strawberries
Sweet potatoes
Swiss chard
Watercress

- **Keep warm.** Basically, anything that helps boost your body temperature also boosts your thyroid function. Sitting in a sauna for ten to twenty minutes, taking a hot bath, sleeping with a down comforter and socks, drinking hot tea instead of ice water—all these simple lifestyle changes can have a big effect.

*   *   *

You may also choose to follow the special thyroid-friendly menu in Part Five as a way to help boost your thyroid's function and avoid goitrogenic foods.

Spying Systemic Yeast

One of the things that can mysteriously and frustratingly prevent us from losing weight is a systemic yeast problem. Most people think of yeast as being vaginal, but everyone has yeast. Yes, men, too. You could have never had an apparent yeast infection in your life and still have yeast overgrowth.

We have a very delicate balance in our gut between friendly flora and yeast. Yeast colonies can rapidly multiply and overtake our friendly flora in response to diet, hormones, or environmental factors. People who eat a lot of sugar are more prone to yeast overgrowth, because yeast feeds on sugar (and thus prompts sugar cravings). Taking antibiotics disturbs your intestinal flora; this is the reason people recommend eating yogurt when you take antibiotics (which really doesn't help much—especially if you are reactive to yogurt!). Other factors that might contribute to yeast overgrowth are hormonal changes, stress, birth control pills, steroids, and exposure to radiation from X-rays or radiation therapy.

Regardless of what causes it, a yeast overgrowth can create digestive disturbances like bloating, gas, constipation, headache, sinus problems, brain fog, depression, and fatigue. Even more, yeast can set off volatile emotional issues. You know all those symptoms usually associated with PMS, like feeling irrational, severe mood swings, and anger? Those can often be a result of systemic yeast, which can increase during times of hormonal shifts. When yeast organisms take over your intestinal flora, they produce acidic toxins, which slow down weight loss and affect your immune system. If you are having a yeast flare-up while testing, it will affect our data. It would be frustrating to put in all this effort on your twenty days and not have the payoff, so we want to determine if there's an issue before we get started.

We use a very easy test for yeast overgrowth. Since yeast feeds on sugar and fermented foods, we do a test day before beginning your Plan on the foods that are the most likely contributors to its growth. Set aside one day and include in your daily menu wine or beer (full of yeasty goodness), balsamic vinegar, and chocolate. Yes, all three in one day; did I mention the test was fun? If you don't drink wine or beer, you can just have the dessert and a heavy dose of balsamic vinegar. If chocolate isn't your thing, you can choose any sweets you love. Keep everything else that day the same as usual. The next morning, upon awakening, check your tongue in the mirror. If it's coated white, it's a sign that yeast is an issue for you.

If it is, don't panic. This is easily treatable. I know there are many hard-core practitioners out there who want to cut from your diet every bit of sugar and everything fermented to control yeast, but I haven't found this strict regimen to be necessary—and frankly, it is pretty depressing. In addition, if the yeast is rampant, this austere approach will cause rapid yeast die-off symptoms, which feel horrible (think extreme detox with foggy thinking and severe moodiness). I believe it's better to let the yeast die off more slowly and, in the meantime, let you enjoy a regular life.

The best way to counteract a yeast overgrowth is through a course of high-quality probiotics. Probiotics are living organisms that are similar to the beneficial bacteria in your stomach that help restore the correct balance in your system. ReNew Life brand is the most effective nationally available line of probiotics we've seen. Choose one that has between 30 and 50 billion active cultures; more than that causes the yeast to die off too rapidly, resulting in the horrible symptoms I mentioned above.

I find that most people respond to probiotic treatment within a week and are ready to start The Plan with yeast issues well under control. You can go ahead and start The Plan after you've taken the probiotics for seven days. You don't need to retest; we'll do this on Day Four, and we'll keep an eye on yeast throughout. If you stay within the guidelines of The Plan, you're very likely not going to have a problem in the future.

Calculating Your Water Intake

Remember me, the one who promised to be the mother you never wanted when it comes to drinking enough water? You're here because you want to get healthy and lose weight, and I'm not going to let something as simple as not drinking the correct amount of water get in your way. Below are the general guidelines for calculating your personal water intake.

How to Calculate Your Daily Water Requirements

- Take your body weight and divide it in half. That is the number of ounces you should be drinking daily.
- For every thirty minutes of cardiovascular exercise you do, add one glass (eight ounces).
- For every forty-five minutes of weight training, add another eight ounces.
- For every glass of wine, add four to six ounces (roughly the equivalent of what you're consuming in alcohol).
- In hot weather, make adjustments similar to exercise (one or two additional glasses, depending on the severity of the heat, how much time you spend outdoors, etc). This is especially important for people who get migraines, because heat can dehydrate you and trigger migraines.
- All teas and your sixteen ounces of a.m. water count toward your daily water intake. Coffee does not count toward your water intake.

Remember, it's essential to get all your water in before dinner, to avoid having it show up the next day on the scale. It's just water weight, yes, but it will still throw off our data. It is easier than you might think to get in all your water during the day. I find it helps to do a mental check-in at noon, 5 p.m., and 7 p.m. If you find yourself short of your recommended amount by dinner, you want to get it in

(continued)

from a health perspective; if your numbers are up the next morning, at least you'll know why.

My client Stephanie, thirty-eight, is a schoolteacher and was worried about the mechanics of drinking that much water during the work day. "It's not that I don't think I can do it," she said. "It's that I only get three breaks a day to leave my classroom." I get it—no one wants to be running to the bathroom all the time! But it's not good to save all your water intake for late in the day, because then you'll be interrupting your sleep cycle to get up during the night to go. I suggested she drink one pint (sixteen ounces) when she first woke up every day, then three more pints spaced throughout the rest of the day. That way the water would run through her system faster and she could time her bathroom breaks. If she was sipping all day long, she'd be sneaking off to the bathroom every half hour.

One last word about water here: drinking more than your recommended amount is not better. In fact, it's almost as detrimental for weight loss as not drinking enough. I've seen this play out over and over: clients overdrink, and they stabilize or gain weight. Your water needs are based on your body mass; drink too much and you stress out your kidneys and retain water. So for all you overachievers out there: more isn't better. Just right is just right.

The Ultimate Prep Tool

Perhaps the most important preparation for The Plan is setting your mind. These twenty days are an investment in yourself. You've worked so hard at other methods that didn't work, and twenty days in comparison is nothing—especially since the information you glean here will give you control over your weight and health *for the rest of your life.*

You deserve this time. You deserve to understand your own body. And most of all, you deserve to look and feel fantastic.

So let's get started.

Susan, 51

I used to have a very unhealthy relationship with food: bad vs good, obsessed with the scale, never fully enjoying what I ate. Binge-ing and guilt were my constant companions.

Until recently. Until going on The Plan. For the first time in my life, I don't even think about these things. I traveled through London and Paris eating what and when I wanted. And it was not a lot. I actually was not that hungry! No cravings. No guilt. No obsession. And when I got home and weighed myself, the number on the scale was a number—*not me*. It was a few pounds, nothing more. No hysteria or obsession: I just went back on The Plan and looked forward to my friendly foods.

The fact that my *head* has changed is the most important benefit. I truly cannot believe it. Before The Plan I was actually considering therapy for healthy eating. Not now. Thank you for giving me back my head.

CHAPTER FOUR

Phase One—The Three-Day Cleanse

Phase One of The Plan is a simple three-day detox. The cleanse resets your body by decreasing inflammation and creating a purified, neutral base line against which you'll begin testing new foods. It gives your system a break from the difficult task of digesting reactive and processed foods, allowing it to return to its natural state of homeostasis.

Right up until the day you die, the body *wants* to renew and repair. That's what it's designed to do. It's truly amazing that way. But when we fill it with foods that are reactive, the body's energy is diverted from a state of homeostasis to the most immediate task at hand (dealing with an "invader") and veers off its intended course. This causes an inflammatory response that can last 72 hours. But when we give it a little nudge by detoxing, it gets right back onto the path of self-healing.

Cleansing the digestive system is a practice that dates back to ancient times. Nearly every culture and religion throughout the centuries recognizes the benefit of detoxifying the body through a cleanse or moderate fast. Lent, Yom Kippur, Ramadan, and Native American vision quests are all times of purification of the soul *and* body. Even Hippocrates promoted the therapeutic value of temporarily taking a break from our everyday eating habits for healing purposes.

The cleanse will also increase your body's sensitivities to foods, which will allow for more accurate testing. Our bodies become desensitized to foods we eat all the time, so it's tough to isolate the ones you're reactive to. This is an advanced form of an elimination/rotation diet, which is typically used to identify food allergies. We remove all but the least reactive foods from your diet for a few days, and then slowly reintroduce one new food at a time to see how your body responds.

Forty-eight-year-old Mara, for example, suffered from chronic constipation and was carrying an extra twenty-five pounds she couldn't lose. She was eating the healthiest foods imaginable, living off 1,200 to 1,500 calories a day, working out with a trainer five days a week, and still not getting anywhere. Like most of my clients, she was incredibly frustrated because her body refused to respond to what used to work for her. Even more, she was really concerned because there was a history of colon cancer in the family, and she was having a bowel movement no more than once a week.

In her initial consultation with me, Mara told me that she loved salmon and ate it close to four nights a week because she felt fantastic eating it. She went on The Plan and was doing great, losing half a pound a day. When you eat foods that aren't inflammatory for you day after day, an amazing thing happens: the body starts to heal. By Day Eight, Mara had lost seven pounds and was starting to have bowel movements regularly. On Day Ten we tested her on her beloved salmon. Ten minutes later, I received a frantic email saying, "My stomach is blowing up like a balloon and my fingers are so swollen that I had to take my rings off!"

The next day, Mara stepped on the scale. Instead of losing the half pound she had been dropping daily since the cleanse, she gained two pounds, and her constipation returned for forty-eight hours. This is a classic reactive response: you eat a low-calorie food, you have exponential weight gain, and whatever is chronic or latent in your health history reappears. Remember, we aren't changing the caloric value of a day by much, so to gain two pounds in one day shows the amazing potency of reactive foods.

Still, Mara was deeply attached to the idea of eating salmon. Like a lot of women, she was really hooked into this ideology that salmon is a superfood that all women over forty need to be eating. So she decided to test it again. We waited a week and got the same response. No question about it: salmon was very clearly reactive for her—and she'd been eating it four nights a week! All we had to do was eliminate salmon as well as her other trigger, eggs, and Mara quickly lost eighteen pounds and has had regular digestion ever since. The upshot here is that had Mara kept right on eating salmon all the way through, we would never have been able to pinpoint it as the inflammatory trigger.

The cleanse also sensitizes something else: your palate. We're going to get out of your diet all the excess salt (hidden in every food that you're not making yourself), which will attune your taste buds to all the other flavors you've been missing. Practically every client I've had is amazed at how salty restaurant food tastes once they've sensitized their palates. Excess sodium causes water retention and exacerbates reactive response to an inflammatory food, so reducing its presence in your system sets you up for better success on The Plan.

Before you begin, I encourage you to read through the menu plans for Days One to Three to familiarize yourself with what's coming and make sure you have all the necessary ingredients on hand. I find it's helpful to prepare as much of the food as possible a day or two beforehand. Many people like to shop on Saturday and prep on Sunday for the entire week, but you can begin anytime that's good for you, as long as you carve out three full days to eat meals that you prepare yourself. To make things easier, we take leftovers from most nights' dinners and use them for lunch the next day. This means less work for you!

To the best of your ability, set aside these three days as time for *you*. If you can, try to do it during a time when you don't have a lot of other big things happening. This is a chance to restore your body at its deepest level and prime it for what will be a life-changing twenty days. Trust that your systems will balance themselves very quickly.

Remember, your body *wants* to renew and repair. Just give it a small break and it will repay you a thousandfold. I have many clients who love the results of the cleanse so much that I actually have to limit how often they repeat it! This is time that you're taking for yourself to reestablish a friendship with your body that you may have lost somewhere along the way.

Lucy, 47

I exercised regularly, ate healthy—or so I thought. I couldn't make the scale budge and had grown used to having stomach issues. The two and a half months that I have spent on The Plan have been fabulous! I lost fifteen pounds. I am not killing myself working out, and the weight is staying off. I very rarely have any stomach issues. And I've gotten everyone in the family hooked on kale! My husband is so amazed at my results that he is starting The Plan in a couple of weeks. Thank you for figuring out this theory of reactive foods. I feel great!

What You Can Expect

There are a lot of intense detox plans out there that are pretty extreme, but I don't believe they're necessary. In fact, they do more harm than good.

Take a juice fast as an example. The body is used to breaking down harmful foods, so when you give it a break, it breathes a sigh of relief and starts to do the repair it naturally wants to do. That's a good thing. The problem is that when you do it in an extreme way and severely limit food or cut it out altogether, your system rapidly releases all the toxins and your organs of elimination get overloaded. Our goal isn't to bombard the body all at once; that would be unkind. Besides the mental torture of severe deprivation, this toxic overload would make you feel pretty awful.

That's why the cleanse we do on The Plan consists of three full meals and a snack. It's important to know that you can detox and lose a lot of weight while still eating real food. The purpose here is to cleanse your system, honor your body's elimination process, *and* stay sane.

Having said that, while the cleanse isn't at all extreme, you're still removing toxins from your system, so there's a chance that some symptoms may show up. As your body purifies itself, you may experience any of the following:

- *Headache.* Double-strength peppermint tea works wonders for headaches. If you feel you need to take a pain reliever, opt for acetaminophen over ibuprofen (ibuprofen is notorious for water retention). Bayer and Excedrin Migraine are also great.
- *Fatigue, lethargy, or weakness.* For many people, their energy levels remain fine, but if you do feel tired, this is an indication that the body has a lot of repair to do. The body repairs best when you sleep. It's exciting when you realize that the body is trying to maximize this cleanse time, and the best remedy is the most obvious one: rest as much as possible and use this time to reflect on your goals.
- *Light-headedness.* Adequate water is essential to combat light-headedness. Emergen-C drink mix, taken one to two times throughout the day, is a great remedy for electrolyte depletion (and muscle cramping as well). Avoid Gatorade, however; it has way too much sodium and sugar. Note that Emergen-C might slow weight loss.
- *Irritability, mild depression, difficulty sleeping.* As the body diverts energy toward repair, other systems and organs can temporarily be affected—including the brain, liver, and nervous system. Studies have shown that SAM-e is an effective liver cleanser and aids the uptake of dopamine, norepinephrine, and serotonin, which decreases depression and anxiety. What I love about SAM-e is that you can take it when you need it and skip it when you don't, without any negative effects.

- *Temporary muscle aches and other flulike symptoms.* Toxins get stored deep in connective tissue, and their release can cause mild achiness. A good remedy for this is taking a hot bath with Epsom salts. Epsom salts contain magnesium sulfate, and since the skin absorbs roughly 65 percent of what is applied topically, they're great for soothing aches and pains (this works well for irritability, too).

- *A coated, pasty tongue.* This is a sign that you had systemic yeast overgrowth. Once again, this is great—your intestinal flora are starting to rebalance. If you see a white coating on your tongue, you can take a good probiotic of 30 to 50 billion cells for a few days to speed up the process.

- *Constipation, diarrhea, or gas.* Again, as your body's energy reserves are tapped for repair, systems like digestion may temporarily be impaired. Ginger, peppermint, or chamomile tea is useful for relief of digestive ailments.

Symptoms such as these are perfectly normal and, thankfully, usually pass within the first twenty-four to forty-eight hours. They are part of what is called the healing crisis, which occurs when the body expels toxins faster than it can eliminate them.

It can come as a bit of a shock to experience detox symptoms if you weren't expecting them. Robert, fifty-one, was a runner and a self-proclaimed health nut. So he was surprised when he felt fatigued and achy two days into the cleanse. He said, "I'm one of the healthiest people I know…I figured I'd sail through the detox, no problem!" I really do understand the frustration of thinking you're eating healthfully, only to discover that your body has been storing toxins as a result of what you're ingesting. But just as I told Robert, I encourage you to recognize that the foods you were eating just weren't healthy for *you*. If you hadn't gone through this healing crisis, you never would have known how much things needed to change.

Try your best to avoid taking any nonessential medications to alleviate symptoms, to give your liver as much of a rest from processing chemicals as possible. Please cut out all supplements if possible, especially fish oil (see sidebar on "The Dangers of Fish Oil"). However, please do not discontinue any prescribed medications without consulting your doctor.

During the cleanse, make sure you drink your recommended daily amount of water to aid your body with elimination. You can also drink unsweetened and noncaffeinated herbal teas. Some people find hot showers helpful, or saunas if they have access to one, as a way of releasing even more toxins through the skin. Calming practices like gentle yoga, slow walks, or meditation can also help center you and make you appreciate how hard your body is working to right itself.

The Dangers of Fish Oil

The Mayo Clinic states that people with fish or shellfish allergies should avoid fish oils. As 85 percent of the people we work with on The Plan are reactive to salmon, taking the oil isn't something I recommend. In addition, fish oils can present other problems, ranging from abnormal liver function to increasing the manic phase of bipolar disorder.

Fish oils can have a damaging effect when combined with certain medications. They can interfere with blood pressure medications and can increase the risk of hemorrhagic stroke and gastrointestinal bleeding in sensitive individuals when combined with blood thinners. Over 25 million Americans suffer from diabetes; fish oils can increase blood sugar and interfere with commonly prescribed medications such as Metformin.

Oils are very sensitive; they go rancid quickly and then become pro-inflammatory. Researchers at New Zealand's Crop and Food Research Institute tested fish oil capsules and found that a large majority of the supplements on the market had already started to go bad long before their expiration dates. One study in Norway (where almost half of the world's fish oils come from) found that 95 percent of the fish oils had started to degrade early on. The study advised that if you burp after taking the supplement—the most common complaint—the oil is rancid and you should discard it immediately.

Are omega-3s important to have as part of our arsenal for health? Absolutely, but first note whether you are reactive to salmon and then discuss with your physician whether taking fish oils may alter the efficacy of your drugs and affect your health. Do not assume that fish oil is a wonder supplement.

Exercising During the Cleanse

While this may surprise you, we recommend *not* working out during the first three days on The Plan. Yes, you read that correctly: no exercising. This is your official permission to take three days off from running, weight lifting, spinning, or whatever you generally do for exercise.

I'm a huge proponent of exercise when it's done right and in healthy moderation. But the cleanse is detox time, when the body's energy needs to be funneled toward repair of its internal systems. If you work out during these crucial days, energy is expended on exercise and then on muscle repair instead of renewing vital organs. Some might think that exercising can only help us lose even more weight, but when we shift our emphasis to what is best for our body for repair, we are always paid back with greater weight loss. You have the rest of your life to work out, so for these three days, *relax*.

In Chapter Five you'll find more information about exercising on The Plan once you're past the first three days.

The Daily Basics of the Cleanse

Beginning on Day One, you'll do two things that will very quickly become your morning routine. The first is to weigh yourself. No dread, no drama. Just step on the scale and record your weight in your Plan Journal. **Remember that your weight is just data**. It's a number that will change and go lower as we begin to root out the foods that are inflammatory triggers for you. This is a daily and methodical exploration to uncover the hidden triggers that have been sabotaging your health, and the scale is simply the instrument you use to collect the necessary information.

The second thing is to drink sixteen ounces of fresh water with a squeeze of lemon juice, and take your liver detox supplement and/or drink a cup of dandelion tea. This liver support is especially crucial during the cleanse, as your body is processing and releasing the toxins built up in your system.

Menu Plans

For each of the twenty days, starting with the cleanse, I'll give you a specific meal plan along with anything and everything you might need to know about the foods being introduced that day. All the foods are tested in a specific order, beginning with the least reactive foods, so the menus are more than just suggestions. You'll want to follow them closely to get the most accurate results possible. Remember, this isn't a diet; it's a testing protocol systematically designed to gather the critical information you need to become the scientific authority on your own body.

We'll get to Day One in just a moment, but first, let me answer some of the most commonly asked questions about the menus:

Can I substitute a food mentioned in a menu plan?

Everything we put into The Plan is carefully chosen—the least reactive foods (and amounts of food) and the most successful combinations—so it's best to stick as close to the menus laid out as possible. Once you go through the twenty days and develop your own template (which you'll learn how to do in Part Three), feel free to start switching things around and adding new foods. But until then, one seemingly innocent deviation can have unintended results that could throw off your testing protocol.

Take fifty-eight-year-old Gloria, who had depression and was also hypothyroid (these two things often go hand in hand). After her first week on The Plan, her depression had abated so markedly that she was planning to taper off her antidepressants. When she told me this news, I was excited for her, and we discussed talking to her doctor as soon as possible.

The next day I received an email from Gloria that said, "I can't get out of bed and I can't stop crying." I was shocked, and we quickly went through her foods from the day before to figure out what had gone wrong. Now I was baffled, because they were all of her friendly foods!

I had Gloria run me through her entire day, step by step. It turned out that she had gone out to dinner and made one small substitution. Instead of ordering broccoli, she'd ordered broccoli rabe. Like a lot of people, Gloria figured that broccoli and broccoli rabe are the same. They aren't. Broccoli rabe is a goitrogenic food that even when cooked may attack thyroid function. In Gloria's case, it was *highly* reactive.

It sounds extreme, but believe me, it can happen. So for now, try to stick to the menu plans as closely as possible so we can judiciously learn what does and doesn't work for your body.

For your snack, however, you can always replace the snack that is listed with fruit (half a piece for women, one whole fruit for men) and a handful of raw nuts or Katie's Kale Chips (recipe on page 211) after Day Four, provided you've tested both already and passed. You can also always replace Homemade Hummus (page 181) with raw almond butter, as long as you've tested okay on almonds.

Do I have to eat the foods listed only at mealtimes?

There's this idea in the dieting world that eating a lot of small meals throughout the day is better. But if we graze all day, we continually divert the body's energy from repair to digestion. I prefer that you eat three meals and a snack and let your body expend its energy on restoring homeostasis.

Can I switch lunch and dinner if I need to?

Yes, you can. You just don't want to switch or pick and choose meals from different days, because the menu plan for each day is chemically balanced. In other words, you can swap Day Six's lunch and dinner, but don't combine Day Six's lunch and Day Five's dinner. Stick with one day's balance of foods.

Some people find they experience an energy dip when they have animal protein for lunch. So if you do swap a dinner and lunch on a day when protein is called for at dinner, pay attention to your energy levels. If you crash in the midafternoon, that's a sign that animal protein at lunch isn't ideal for you. Do not have soup at dinner time. However, you can have sautéed vegetables instead.

Can I drink coffee?

We eliminate coffee during the cleanse in order to give your liver a chance to fully detox. I have nothing against coffee; it tastes great, is a terrific antioxidant, and is very emotionally satisfying. But it is mildly stressful on the liver, which as you already know is a key organ in over five hundred functions, including detoxification and hormonal control. So if you can make it through just three days and give your liver a little extra love, the payoff will be sizable.

If you think caffeine withdrawal might be an issue, try starting the day with green or black tea (but please limit yourself to two cups because of acid levels, which can set your day off on an inflammatory note). A nice cup of English Breakfast tea could have 70 to 80 milligrams of caffeine, which is just shy of the amount in a cup of coffee.

Having said that, I know coffee is a big one for a lot of people. And I'll tell you the same thing I tell my clients: if you're really miserable without your morning cup, by all means go ahead and have it (but please, no decaf, as it is often made from beans that are more acidic). I'm not going to tell you not to. You're the boss here. It's simply a question of what level of commitment you're looking to make to yourself and your body. Will The Plan work if you don't give up coffee? Yes. Will the detox be much more effective if you do? No question about it. (Note: If you suffer from acid reflux, coffee—especially decaf—will exacerbate acid. Darker roasts, like French Roast, are less acidic and a better choice.)

Can I add spices or condiments?

Feel free to add any of the following anti-inflammatory spices and seasonings whenever you wish:

Basil
Black pepper
Cardamom
Cayenne
Cinnamon
Cloves
Cumin
Garlic
Ginger
Maine Coast Sea Seasonings
Nutmeg
Onion
Oregano
Rosemary
Thyme
Turmeric

The spices you want to avoid are paprika, licorice, chili powder, and fennel, as they may exacerbate inflammation. Additionally, avoid seasoning mixes that contain MSG, which triggers inflammation. By law, seasoning manufacturers are not required to disclose whether they include MSG, so steer clear of any spice mix that just says "spices" without listing the individual ingredients.

During the cleanse, please refrain from adding salt to your food. Remember, we're looking to decrease your sodium intake to sensitize your palate, reduce sugar cravings, and create a noninflammatory base line in your system. Maine Coast Sea Seasonings, seaweed-based seasonings, are an excellent alternative to salt that many of my clients adopt forever purely because they love them. After Day Four, sea salt may be used in moderation. Sea salt, as opposed to table salt and kosher salt, contains eighty minerals that help to metabolize the sodium.

In terms of condiments, please avoid mustard entirely until you have tested it, as it can be highly reactive. I've seen clients gain a pound and have migraines triggered just from a few tablespoons of coarse-grain mustard. Ketchup can be a problem, too, and isn't part of The Plan. But don't worry—we have plenty of sauces to keep you happy.

What about butter? During the cleanse, we take a break from butter to give our digestive system a rest, but after Day Four: absolutely! In fact, butter is an excellent source of many essential vitamins and minerals, most notably vitamin D. (Please see the sidebar for more about butter.) When you add fat to a grain carbohydrate, it slows down the absorption of sugars. Having dry toast without butter is like asking to gain weight. So once you've tested foods like bread, potatoes, and more, slather on the butter and enjoy.

The Redemption of Butter

For years, butter has been vilified, but this delicious spread actually contains many important fat-soluble vitamins and trace minerals that can be otherwise hard to get: vitamin D (which aids calcium absorption and hormonal balance), vitamin E (a powerful antioxidant), zinc (for immunity), and copper (helpful for inflammatory diseases like rheumatoid arthritis and inflammatory bowel disease, or IBD). Butter has more selenium per gram than wheat germ (selenium is very difficult to find in our diet and is essential for thyroid health and immunity).

The big concern for years about butter was that it would raise cholesterol, but most of the theories about the link between fat and cholesterol were actually debunked by the Food and Drug Administration back in 2003. If you think about it, how can so many people be on low-fat diets for cholesterol with no effect? Many other factors go into creating high cholesterol, including a high-glycemic diet and genetics.

Everyone got on the "fat is bad" bandwagon, but what we really need to worry about are trans fats. Those are the fats found in highly processed foods like donuts, packaged cakes and cookies, fried foods, frozen dinners, and more. Anything that lists partially hydrogenated oils in its ingredients contains trans fat, even if it lists 0% on the label (food manufacturers can manipulate portion sizes to sneak that labeling in under the wire, but don't be fooled!). Trans fats not only raise our LDLs (harmful cholesterols), they actually lower our HDL levels (the good cholesterol that our body needs) and are suspected of affecting our body's ability to use important omega-3 fatty acids. The good news here: butter is not a trans fat!

While we're on the topic of cholesterol, let's address the myth that fats raise cholesterol. *Any* food that doesn't work with your chemistry has the potential to raise cholesterol. Remember that inflammation is the culprit behind all disease and all health issues. If you eat a food that is inflammatory for you, it will trigger whatever is latent in your system—including high cholesterol. Oatmeal is revered as a superfood that lowers cholesterol, and if it's friendly for you, there's a good chance it will do that. But if you are reactive to it—which 85 percent of people are—it will actually raise your cholesterol. Same for skim milk and green beans. Again and again, the underlying factor is always reactivity and inflammation.

So given that butter is low reactive, contains no trans fats, includes nutrients that are lacking in our diet, helps with satiety, and tastes delicious, by all means go ahead and enjoy it!

For the first three days, please stick to olive oil with lemon juice and herbs for salad dressing. Beginning on Day Four, feel free to use one of the salad dressing recipes in Part Four. Or if you want to use a premade dressing after Day Four, please choose one with a sodium content limited to 7 percent or less of the RDA (recommended daily allowance) per two-tablespoon serving and whose ingredients you can pronounce. Throughout The Plan, please avoid ranch, blue cheese, or any other dressing that contains dairy until you have tested it. (I'll admit to having a personal gripe against blue cheese, which is injected with mold. You wouldn't want mold in your house, so why do you want it in your body?) And, of course, no dressings that contain mustard until you've tested it. Many balsamic vinaigrettes have mustard in them, so be sure to read the labels carefully.

Many people ask about sugar and other sweeteners. Sugar itself, within reason, is fine. But no, no, no to aspartame and all its friends! These toxic chemicals, called excitotoxins, latch on to brain cells and shorten their life-span. In addition, excitotoxins cause sugar cravings and water retention. Diseases like Alzheimer's and neurological disorders like Parkinson's have been linked to artificial sweeteners. I encourage you to avoid any sugar-free products now and forever. Sugarless gum is not recommended, either. Not only does it contain aspartame, but it causes digestive disorders. You're chewing and setting your body up to digest food that never arrives, which only increases hunger. Additionally, we have found that even "natural" sugar substitutes such as Stevia slow down weight loss, so we do not recommend its use.

Sugar itself (within reason) is fine. Don't worry about sugar. Would honey or agave nectar be better? Yes, but at the end of the day, it's not going to make a huge difference. The body is going to burn foods that aren't chemically processed in a much cleaner way. The more chemically processed something is, the more work it takes for the body to digest it, and then we start to slow down other bodily functions as a result of siphoning off all that energy.

Do I have to eat everything listed on a particular day?

We're all so programmed to think that less is more when it comes to weight loss, but that couldn't be further from the truth. Remember, it's about chemistry, not calories.

People often tell me they can't finish all the food on The Plan— and this is during the cleanse! All the meals in The Plan are chemically balanced to give your body the nutrients it needs and to ensure that you feel satisfied. Skipping any part of a meal will very likely have the opposite effect from what you intend. You'll end up famished later and will overeat, or your body will hold on to weight because it senses it is going into starvation mode.

A classic mistake many people make is to cut out the fat in their diet. You need fat! The brain is 60 percent fat, and it needs fat to function. So do our cells. Our cell walls have a phospholipid barrier, which is a layer of protection containing fatty acids that is sustained through the ingestion of good fats. Without that protective layer, our cell walls become permeable and we become susceptible to free radicals that lead to cancer, autoimmune diseases, and more. Plus, fat satiates you. The more full-fat foods you have in a meal, the less you'll be reaching for snacks later on. One client of mine kept saying she was hungry every day after lunch, even though she was eating great big salads, cooked vegetables, and protein. I finally figured out that it was because she refused to put olive oil on her salads. The day she finally poured it on, she was full all afternoon.

Don't be shy with the olive oil, butter, cheese, and nuts once you pass those tests—especially in the winter, when the body subconsciously craves more fattening foods to sustain us through the cold weather. It's a basic biological response that kept us around after many other species went extinct, so there has to be something to it.

The other important requirement each day is protein. You don't need to do any calculating for now, since all the meals are carefully calibrated for you. But in case you're curious, we have the protein needs for the day structured. For women you're having 10 to 40 grams for breakfast (15 to 60 for men), 15 to 25 grams for lunch (20 to 40 for men), and 25 to 40 grams for dinner (40 to 65 for men). This is actually a very high-protein diet, but unlike traditional high-protein diets, it's high in vegetarian protein, which is easier for your body to digest and essential for repair.

Skimping on protein or fat impedes weight loss. Really. I mean it. I really do. In fact, by not following these guidelines and just having vegetables and fruit, you will cause weight gain or stabilization—and get extremely frustrated. How many people do you know who are just having salads and finding that the weight won't budge? So please, enjoy all the foods listed on the menu plans, and eat until you are full. If you truly are too full to eat everything listed, simply cut down on the portion sizes, but be sure to incorporate at least some of each food listed for that meal to maintain the right chemical balance.

What if I get hungry between meals?

Since the portion sizes are generous and all of your nutritional requirements are easily met on The Plan, it's highly unlikely that you'll be hungry. If you are, the first question to ask yourself is whether you are genuinely eating until you're full.

If you are in fact eating until you are full and still feel hungry, take a look at your daily water intake and see if you have fallen off your mark. Dehydration is often masked as hunger, so your body may actually be signaling that you need water rather than food. As ancient gatherers, it was easier for human beings to find plants than a running body of water. When we needed water, we would grab a berry or a piece of fruit. Biologically, as we evolved, this created some confusion in the switchboard of signals, so our brain registers "find food" when really it means "get water."

If the additional water does not satiate your hunger, you can increase the portion size of your vegetables (larger portions of protein and fruits are tests, which we can carry out later).

Will I crave sweets and other foods I'm used to eating?

The short answer to this, as long as you're eating all the foods listed each day, is no. When your days are nutritionally balanced, you'll probably find yourself marveling that you're not experiencing any cravings. Even the most die-hard pizza and ice cream fans have told me that they barely think about pizza or ice cream after the first week. Does this mean you'll never have foods like that again? Of course not. This is not a restrictive diet. Wine, cheese, bread, and desserts are all encouraged! We are just systematically testing them and then adding them in when they work for you. It's all based on what you love and what you miss most.

If you do find that you are having sugar cravings, there's a chance it's because you're experiencing some yeast die-off symptoms. Be sure to check your tongue in the mornings to see if it is coated white; that's a classic sign of yeast overgrowth. This is where probiotics will come in very handy. When yeast die off, they "trick" your body into feeding them sugar, which helps the colony regrow. This yeast die-off will also trigger anxiety and hormonal disorders, so let's take care of it immediately with probiotics and by avoiding fermented products like vinegar and beer until the yeast is under control.

A lot of times, I've found that increasing fat intake will decrease sugar cravings. You can try adding a little more olive oil, or using an extra tablespoon of raw almond butter, or sprinkling extra seeds on your salad. That usually does the trick!

Flavorful tea like peppermint, rooibos, or chamomile can also be helpful. Unfortunately, the primary flavors we've become accustomed to are sugar and salt, but there's a whole wide world of wonderful tastes out there. Clean and healthy doesn't mean flavorless. In fact, people on The Plan tell me they have never eaten food that is so flavorful. Don't be afraid to explore your spice cabinet; there are also many salt-free blends that you can experiment with.

If none of these work and the sugar cravings are too intense, you can take a supplement called L-glutamine for a short period. Research shows that it is effective in decreasing sugar cravings. It also helps to convert fat into lean muscle mass and is excellent for many chronic digestive disorders such as Crohn's disease. You can start with the commonly recommended dosage of 1,000 milligrams, to be taken at night. As with any supplement, I recommend taking L-glutamine only as long as you need to. Once the cravings subside, you can stop taking it and allow your body's natural regulators to take over. Very often this happens as quickly as a few days.

L-glutamine is a very useful tool to have in your arsenal. My client Naomi, thirty-seven, had intense sugar cravings that she got under control on The Plan. She's an accountant, and every year during tax season she would get so stressed that she would revert to sugar. This would trigger her underlying systemic yeast problem, and she'd spiral into even more sugar cravings. Thinking ahead, we decided to have her start taking L-glutamine and probiotics two weeks before tax season. We both laughed at the simplicity of this suggestion, but it worked. It's better to be proactive about your body's needs instead of trying to grit your teeth and bear it. If you know for certain that you're going to be stressed out and have that sugar response, work with it. Don't try to brush off the stressors in your life. That's where people run into a problem. If you know that during times of high stress you reach for sugar, simply plan for it!

It's the same for a multivitamin. If you know you're going to be going through a particularly busy time and won't be able to eat correctly, then by all means, add in a multivitamin preemptively. Once the intense period is past, you can go right back to relying on good food as your best medicine. Please note that L-glutamine can cause water retention.

Cooking on The Plan

As I mentioned, it's best to familiarize yourself with the menus and recipes for Days One to Three and to prepare as much as possible beforehand. You don't want to wake up on Day One and have to scramble to get what you need.

For the cleanse and throughout The Plan, I recommend preparing as many foods in big batches as possible. For instance, whip up a large pot of Carrot Ginger Soup (page 295), some of which you'll have on Day One, and then freeze the rest for days to come (this is your go-to soup when you're reactive, to calm inflammation). Or cook a batch of chicken on Day Three to keep in the fridge; you can then add the sauces and toppings each day as needed.

All of the recipes on The Plan are easy to follow, even for kitchen beginners. I've had people come to me who couldn't do much more than scramble an egg. By the time they've gone through The Plan, they're amazed by how easy and simple Plan-friendly meals are to prepare—and how delicious they taste. My client Harley recently emailed me to say that she'd gone on vacation with two other families and followed Plan guidelines while she was away. Half the time she dined out and half the time she made Plan-friendly meals. Her friends couldn't stop talking about how much they loved the Plan-friendly meals (and Harley lost three pounds on vacation!).

I'm often asked about organic versus nonorganic produce, and here's my take on that. Of course, it's always best to get the highest-quality foods that you can, and often that means organic. But I also know that's not always possible, or economical, so I tell clients to try to stick to organic just for what's known as the Dirty Dozen. The Dirty Dozen was established by the Environmental Working Group (EWG), a non-profit organization whose mission is to protect public health and the environment. The Dirty Dozen is a list of the fruits and vegetables with the highest pesticide residue: apples, celery, sweet bell peppers, peaches, strawberries, nectarines (imported), grapes, spinach, lettuce, cucumbers, blueberries (domestic), and potatoes (in 2012, the EWG created a Dirty Dozen Plus category, as well, to include green beans and kale/collard greens).

As for chicken and meat, you don't have to buy organic if it's too expensive for your budget, but do try to find hormone-and antibiotic-free. When you compare costs, you might find that you are in fact spending the same amount of money because you're using smaller portions. Plus, you are getting the bonus of more nutritious food that is ethically raised, and there's much value in that. But overall, unless you have a compromised immune system, organic versus nonorganic rarely has a dramatic effect on your body's response to testing a food.

Steaming and sautéing are always the healthiest ways to cook, followed by roasting and grilling. I recommend water sautéing, using herbs and spices or even juice. As soon as the food is cooked, you can add your olive oil. The goal here is not to cut down on the oil, but to maximize its health benefits (oils degrade when they are heated past their set point). Any recipes listed in Part Four of this book where sautéing in olive oil is called for can all be water sautéed as well.

All meats and fish can be sautéed, broiled, or baked. With the exception of chicken, rare to medium-rare works best, as the proteins and fats in meats are unstable when heated and may affect your response if overcooked. (In fact, if you test reactive to salmon, you might want to re-test with salmon sashimi. Same with beef: if you usually have your steak well done and don't pass the beef test, try beef carpaccio.) When you cook protein, the protein molecules are unfolded by the heat. This is called denaturing. Physical and chemical changes occur—some of which are beneficial, but many of which are not! When the fats in protein are exposed to high heat, they develop free radicals, which are inflammatory by nature. Meats cooked at high temperatures (like barbecued meat) have even been found to be carcinogenic. So try not to overcook your proteins.

Roasting vegetables releases their natural sugars, which is what makes them so delicious. You want to keep an eye on the sugar levels, though, which is why in our twenty-day menu plans we recommend limiting roasted vegetables to one or two cups a day as a start. After that, you can find your own balance.

Portions on The Plan

One of the things you'll notice on The Plan is that it's not based on portion sizes. Remember, it's never about counting calories, or weighing your food, or anything like that! Throughout the menu plans, you will see only a small handful of foods for which portion sizes are listed; when there *is* a portion size, it's designed to minimize any reactivity potential of those foods and mitigate excess sugar (which triggers yeast overgrowth). For everything else, you can use the general Plan guidelines below. You may be able to tolerate more or less, and soon you'll come up with your own template, which will work best for your body.

- **Animal protein:** One serving is 4 to 6 ounces for women and 6 to 8 ounces for men (about the size of the palm of each gender's hand, respectively).

- **Vegetables**: Unless otherwise indicated (like for roasted vegetables, which are naturally higher in sugar), please feel free to eat Plan-friendly cooked vegetables until you feel full.
- **Salads**: Eat until you feel full.
- **Soups**: Eat until you feel full.
- **Cheese**: We have found 1 ounce to be the optimal amount to begin with.
- **Nuts and seeds**: When they're included in salads or eaten as a snack, please use a generous handful (unless otherwise indicated), which is roughly 1 ounce for women and 1½ ounces for men.

The Plan for Day One

Day One is the most basic day on The Plan and incorporates only the least reactive foods.

UPON AWAKENING

- Weigh yourself and record the results in your Plan Journal.
- Drink 16 ounces of fresh water with lemon juice (after you weigh yourself).
- Take your liver support supplement and/or drink a cup of dandelion tea.

BREAKFAST

For women: 1 cup of flax granola with ½ cup of blueberries
For men: 1½ cups of flax granola with 1 cup of blueberries
Silk coconut milk or Rice Dream

LUNCH

Carrot Ginger Soup (page 178) with chia seeds or sunflower seeds
Sautéed or steamed broccoli drizzled with Orange Oil (page 176) and lemon juice (make enough to have some left over for lunch on Day Two)

Mixed greens with ½ a medium-sized pear and a handful of
  pumpkin seeds

SNACK

1 medium-sized apple

DINNER

Sautéed Kale with Vegetables (page 178) with Spicy Coco Sauce
  (page 177) (make enough to have some left over for dinner
  on Day Two)
Beet and Carrot Salad (page 178) with pumpkin seeds

WATER

Be sure to drink your recommended daily water intake throughout the day, ending before dinner.

The Inside Scoop on Day One

I include the flax granola every morning during the cleanse for a few
reasons. Flaxseeds are rich in omega-3s and calcium. They are also
loaded with protein—they pack 40 grams into just one cup—which
is an important component of breakfast for satiety, energy, and repair.

As you'll probably find out very quickly, the flax granola is pretty
magical. It is excellent for digestion and even better for elimination.
Whole flaxseeds are soaked overnight so they can release mucilage
(a tasteless gel-like substance); this is what does an internal sweep
in your intestines. If constipation has traditionally been a problem
for you, this will be your best friend and especially helpful since
you're eliminating coffee, which increases peristalsis (the contraction
of muscles through the digestive tract that stimulates elimination).

Lastly, many people are used to and enjoy eating cereal in the
morning. If a bowl of crunchy cereal is what starts your day off on a
happy note, then that's what you should be able to have. The overall
goal here is to develop an eating plan that works not just for your

body, but for your lifestyle—and your sense of satisfaction from what you eat is a big part of that.

It's important to choose whole flaxseeds for your granola rather than ground seeds. Flaxseeds have estrogenic properties, and too much creates hormonal imbalance. When the flaxseeds are ground, your body will absorb more of these estrogenic properties; keeping them whole cuts down that absorption significantly.

You can order flax granola directly from Columbia County Bread (www.columbiacountybread.com), or very easily make it yourself by following the recipe on page 173. Most people like the nutty taste of the granola, but if it doesn't quite resonate with your palate at first, give it a few days. You'll be amazed at how quickly your taste buds will change and adjust to foods that are healthier. Adding some extra raisins or cinnamon can boost the flavor, as does using vanilla-flavored rice milk or coconut milk. And by the way, cinnamon is excellent for aiding digestion, controlling type 2 diabetes, lowering cholesterol, and helping decrease arthritic pain, so there's an added health benefit to sprinkling it on.

After the first week on The Plan, we start to rotate in alternate breakfasts, as the body adapts to stimulus and you start to lose a positive response (in fact, all foods are best rotated to maximize their health benefits). After twenty days, you'll want to try to limit the flax granola to twice a week for maximum health benefits (and yes, it really gets that addictive!).

Lastly, a quick note about the Spicy Coco Sauce. This sauce is a major Plan favorite (I've had clients say it's so good that they would eat kitty litter if it had Spicy Coco Sauce on it), so you might want to make a little extra and freeze it to use in days to come. Some clients like to freeze their Spicy Coco Sauce in ice cube trays to make individual portions and then just add it to their sautés as desired for extra flavor.

The first day of your cleanse, you may feel a little fatigued. Yes, repair can start this quickly! This is a good sign. If your body is trying to make you shut down and sleep, it's communicating with you loud and clear to hit the hay and let it do some deep repair work. It's amazing how badly your body wants to heal, so let it.

Day One is a great time to schedule a little personal pampering to help your body in its restoration process. If you can, go for a long walk, meditate, schedule a massage, take a sauna, or just make a plan to watch a favorite movie, read a good book, or enjoy some quality time with people who matter to you. The goal is to restore and nourish yourself, inside and out.

The Plan for Day Two

Day Two incorporates your first "test," which is almonds. It's essential that you choose raw, unsalted almonds to get the most accurate reading. Roasted nuts, while delicious, are much higher in reactivity, so for now we'll stick with raw to determine how your body responds. If you find you gain weight or are reactive to almonds in any way, you'll omit them from your menu going forward. You can always try low-reactive nut butters instead, such as sunflower butter.

Raw vs Roasted Nuts

If you heat oil beyond its set point, the oil's chemical structure changes. When you do that and you're in an inflammatory state, it can provoke an inflammatory reaction. Most people find raw nuts that work for them, but commercially roasted nuts are more than 80 percent reactive (meaning that they are reactive for more than 80 percent of our clientele; we'll talk more about reactivity levels of specific foods in Chapter Five). Most nuts are roasted at high heat in oils that contain trans fats with a lower set point. Then a roasted nut can sit on a shelf, causing rancidity. All that is to say: raw nuts are a far friendlier choice. If you love roasted nuts, there will be plenty of chances to test them later on—or you can roast them yourself.

UPON AWAKENING

- Weigh yourself and record the results in your Plan Journal.
- Drink 16 ounces of fresh water with lemon juice (after you weigh yourself).
- Take your liver support supplement and/or drink a cup of dandelion tea.

BREAKFAST

For women: 1 cup of flax granola with ½ cup of blueberries
For men: 1½ cups of flax granola with 1 cup of blueberries
Silk coconut milk or Rice Dream

LUNCH

Carrot Ginger Soup (page 178) with sunflower seeds
Mixed greens with ½ diced apple and ¼ avocado
Leftover broccoli from Day One

SNACK

For women: ½ pear with a small handful of almonds
For men: 1 pear with a small handful of almonds

DINNER

For women: Leftover Sautéed Kale with Vegetables with 1 cup of
   basmati rice and pumpkin seeds
For men: Leftover Sautéed Kale with Vegetables with 1½ cups of
   basmati rice and pumpkin seeds
Beet and Carrot Salad (page 178) with sunflower seeds

WATER

Be sure to drink your recommended daily water intake throughout the day, ending by 7:30 p.m.

The Inside Scoop on Day Two

Rice is a very low-reactive grain, which is why we introduce it so
early on in The Plan. Brown rice is high in fiber but also high in
arsenic; basmati rice is always a better choice. A lot of clients email
me to say that it's been years since they've had rice, so go ahead and
enjoy!

The Plan for Day Three

Today you'll be introducing chickpeas (in the Spicy Vegetarian Soup,
page 180), which are a nice source of protein and an easy gateway
test for the legume family. Canned chickpeas are fine; just be sure
to choose the low-sodium variety that has less than 100 milligrams.
Remember that sodium exacerbates reactivity and impedes weight
loss, so this is important. Simply getting the regular kind and rinsing
them, as many people do, won't work because the chickpeas are permeable and are submerged in the salty solution for months.

UPON AWAKENING

- Weigh yourself and record the results in your Plan Journal.
- Drink 16 ounces of fresh water with lemon juice (after you
  weigh yourself).
- Take your liver support supplement and/or drink a cup of dandelion tea.

BREAKFAST

For women: 1 cup of flax granola with choice of ½ cup of blueberries or ½ diced pear

For men: 1 cup of flax granola with choice of 1 cup of blueberries or 1 whole pear
Silk coconut milk or Rice Dream

LUNCH

Baby romaine lettuce with ¼ avocado, pumpkin seeds, and carrots
Spicy Vegetarian Soup (page 180) with ½ cup of low-sodium
chickpeas added

SNACK

For women: 10 to 12 raw almonds (if you tested reactive to
almonds yesterday, you can replace this with ½ apple or pear)
For men: 18 raw almonds (can be replaced with 1 whole apple or
pear)

DINNER

For women: 2 to 3 ounces of Chicken with Italian Herbs and
Orange Zest (page 182) on a bed of mixed greens
For men: 4 ounces of Chicken with Italian Herbs and Orange Zest
(page 182) on a bed of mixed greens
Roasted Italian Winter Vegetables (page 184; 1 cup for women, 2
cups for men; make enough to have some left over for dinner
on Day Four)

The Inside Scoop on Day Three

There are a few things worth knowing about chicken as it relates to
The Plan. The first is that it's universally the least reactive animal protein, which is why we include it so early on and it doesn't count as a
"test." While I don't like to make absolute statements, I can say that
pretty much everyone loses weight on chicken.

The second thing that's helpful to know is that nearly everyone loses weight on chicken *as long as it's not prepared at a restaurant.* The interesting fact about chicken is that when it's prepared by a food establishment, it's usually loaded with sodium. Restaurants add salt for flavoring, and the tricky part is that chicken hides the taste so well that we can easily and unknowingly consume three times the amount of recommended sodium in one dish. Even those plain roasted chicken breasts you buy at the supermarket that look so innocent are likely cooked in chicken broth, which is packed with sodium and MSG (a huge trigger for weight gain and headaches). Of course, it never hurts to test something prepared at a grocery store, like rotisserie chicken, for ease of preparation or if that's something you normally eat and enjoy. Once you know how to test, you can use this simple method that I suggest to my clients: take off half the skin and drizzle the chicken with lemon or lime juice to help offset the sodium. Weigh yourself the next day and see if your grocery store passes the test!

The regular portion size for animal protein on The Plan is 4 to 6 ounces for women and 6 to 8 ounces for men, which is about the size of the palm of each gender's hand, respectively. On Day Three, we reintroduce animal protein slowly to ease out of the detox, which is why we do a half portion of chicken. Going forward, you'll increase to the larger portion size, and then if you want to test a bigger portion at some point, you can do so. Again, everything is a test—including larger portion sizes than we include during these twenty days.

On Day Three we also include roasted vegetables. Roasting vegetables releases their natural sugars, which is why they're so delicious. Eating too many roasted vegetables, however, overloads your system with sugar. Natural sugar is still sugar, which—if you overdo it—can aggravate underlying systemic yeast, affect glucose levels, or impede weight loss. That's also why it's so important to always have a salad with your cooked vegetable, so you have a mix of vegetables. In addition, the enzymes in the raw vegetables from the salad aid digestive function.

In warmer weather, you may be able to eat just raw vegetable salads alone, but once we get into winter, too many cold, raw vegetables in your system will hamper digestion (which is why so many people who are eating just salads all winter long are wondering why they feel bloated). As a general rule of thumb, in colder temperatures, aim to keep a good ratio of cooked and raw vegetables on your plate. Once summer rolls around, you can feel free to cut back on the cooked vegetables and see how you do.

Ending Your Cleanse

With the chicken dinner on Day Three, your cleanse officially comes to an end. Starting tomorrow, you'll begin Phase Two—the testing phase. Life gets back to normal and you'll be enjoying things like coffee, cheese, chocolate, wine, and more. You've done a great job flushing toxins from your system, reducing inflammation, and priming your body beautifully for the testing days ahead.

Alison, 43

The Plan changed my life. Really.

Prior to finding out about The Plan, I had just about given up hope that my weight would ever be different than what it was. I was certainly not obese, but I was at least thirty to forty pounds overweight. Over the past four to five years, I had gained weight steadily to a number that I never thought I'd see on the scale. I tried several diet plans to lose the weight. Each time, I would see some moderate success, and then life would get in the way and I would give up.

As someone who prided herself on eating healthy, I would have Greek yogurt and peanut butter for breakfast. The problem became the rest of the day. For lunch, I would have whatever was in the kitchen. And dinner was not that much better. As a mom who makes several meals for the family, I would cook healthy for the kids and

(continued)

my husband and then just eat cereal or pasta—whatever would "fill me up." Then I'd have sweet binges in the evening. Whether it was chocolate or some sort of candy, I would eat until I had satisfied the craving. That would result in poor sleep and then a difficult next day. I was short with my family, my hair was thinning, and I was often having histamine reactions, during which my nose would run after eating foods that I deemed healthy. Overall, I felt pretty mediocre.

I'd pile on the exercise, as I naturally thought the more I did, the more weight I would lose. So in addition to three days a week of boot camp, I worked out one day with a personal trainer. I played tennis and I even trained for a triathlon. It was all done in the name of more is better for losing weight.

Once I read about The Plan in a magazine, something clicked. Everything Lyn-Genet spoke about resonated with me in such a real and personal way that I knew this was the plan for me. I loved that The Plan was providing me with a blueprint of foods that I could count on to make me healthy. Being the CEO of my family, I needed to have "go-to foods" that I could eat that I wouldn't have to think too much about but know they were good for my body and my weight loss goals.

The Plan made me more aware of things I already knew. For example, I always knew that water was important, but I didn't have a full appreciation of _how_ important. I know now that if I don't hydrate enough, particularly in the morning, I'll be craving salty food by midafternoon. For years I couldn't get my rings off my fingers. My "aha" came after a week on The Plan, when I could suddenly get my rings off at night. I also connected the dots and realized that my sweet cravings hit whenever I had ingested a lot of sodium. Learning to truly listen to your body is life altering.

There are many things that I had to "unlearn." For example, we're always told that potato chips are bad for you. What we should be told instead is that regular salty potato chips are bad for you—but _unsalted_ potato chips help to stave off a reaction to sodium. In fact, last week I was concerned that my dinner was too salty, so right after,

I had about ten unsalted potato chips and two glasses of red wine. Lost weight that night!

And exercise—boy, did I have that wrong. Not only was I not losing weight with my overabundance of exercise, but I was probably gaining weight. I no longer feel the need to "pile it on" to lose weight, as my current pared-down regimen of four times a week is just fine.

I love that one of the keys to success on The Plan is variety. In fact, at one point, I was having chicken so many days in a row and was getting bored. The Plan encourages you to mix up your proteins, which will help with weight loss. I also love how Lyn-Genet says that when you gain weight from a food, it's not that you were bad—it's that your body is trying to tell you something and you need to listen.

In just seven short months, I've lost close to twenty pounds. My hair has gotten thicker and longer. I have stopped sniffling after most meals and the patches of eczema on my knees have diminished. I feel so amazing and energized. People have said that I'm glowing. When they ask me about my diet, I explain that it's not a diet—it's a change in the way I eat. I have always enjoyed cooking, but now I have such an appreciation for making fresh food instead of canned or jarred (even if it's organic prepared sauces). I still haven't quite mastered preparing sauces and dressings ahead of time so I'm not struggling at the last moment, but I'll get there. That's the beauty of The Plan: you can do it on your own time. It's a constant work in progress. And as our body continues to change, we need to as well.

CHAPTER FIVE

Phase Two—The Testing Phase

Nancy, 40

I often gain weight when I "disconnect" from myself. But The Plan required me to stay connected. I deliberately observed how my body reacted to food, and that has helped me tremendously. Each morning I measured my weight loss and reported how I felt. If I experienced a reaction (fatigue, headache, weight gain), I learned how to use the data to plan accordingly. I lost eighteen pounds the first month I implemented The Plan. I stopped all cravings. I was a big diet soda drinker, and I no longer desire it. The Plan helped me learn what foods are friendly for my system and what foods I should limit. Most of all, I no longer "disconnect." The Plan has given me back a real relationship with my body.

Now that you've created a neutral base line within your body, you're ready to begin Phase Two of The Plan: the testing stage. Just like in the cleanse, we're going to start with the friendliest foods first and slowly work our way up to more potentially problematic foods. We want to be as kind to your body as possible and not start off with foods that have a higher chance of compromising your health or weight.

This reactive food list is based on years of hands-on experience, research, and collection of data—not unlike what you're about to do for your own body, except you'll have it down in a matter of weeks, not years. My staff and I have worked with thousands of clients, and every day we continually monitor and record their responses to specific foods. The chart below covers the reactivity potential of many of the most common foods, based on this research. The rates refer to the percentage of our clientele that tested reactive to that food.

Reactive Foods

85% + Reactive
- Shrimp
- Turkey
- Tomato sauce
- Eggplant
- Oatmeal
- Greek yogurt
- Black beans
- Cannellini beans
- Cauliflower
- Cabbage
- Hard-boiled eggs
- Non-organic spinach
- Salmon
- Asparagus
- Bagels
- Farm-raised fish
- Corn
- Sushi
- Deli meats

70% Reactive
- Yogurt, regular
- Green beans
- Pork
- Pasta
- Bananas
- Roasted nut butter
- Walnuts

- Strawberries
- Veal
- Green peppers

60% Reactive
- Red peppers
- Mushrooms (excluding shiitake)
- Cod
- Tuna
- Pineapple
- Grapefruit
- Artichokes
- Quinoa
- Oranges
- Melons (except watermelon)

50% Reactive
- Cow's milk
- Couscous
- White rice
- Almond milk
- Tomatoes
- Edamame
- Whole eggs
- Tahini

40% Reactive
- Wild white fish
- Lentils
- Peas
- Lactose-free milk
- Egg whites

30% Reactive
- Bok choy
- Cow's cheese
- Brussels sprouts

20% Reactive
- Wheat
- Scallops
- Snow peas
- Winter squash
- Crab
- Sashimi
- Spelt
- Kamut
- Sesame seeds
- Tempeh

10% Reactive
- Potatoes (in small amounts)
- Duck
- Hemp seeds

(continued)

5% or Less Reactive
- Pit fruits *(mangoes, avocadoes, etc.)*
- Garlic
- Chickpeas
- Onions
- Shiitaki mushrooms *(may be higher if you have systemic yeast)*
- Radicchio
- Lamb
- Chicken
- Goat or sheep's cheese
- Pears
- Broccoli
- Carrots
- Kale
- Zucchini
- Beets
- Steak
- Sunflower seeds
- Pumpkin seeds
- Raw almonds
- Apples
- Pears
- Blueberries
- Rice cereal
- Chia seeds
- Frisee
- Coconut milk
- Rice milk

While the list may seem daunting at first glance, all that matters is *your* response to food. If you've been unknowingly eating one of your personal triggers for years, your list of personally reactive foods may be longer initially because your body is in an inflamed state. The good news is that when you lower your chronic low-grade inflammation, there is a good chance that you will then be able to enjoy these foods on a regular basis.

The Devil Foods

There's reactive, and then there's wildly reactive. Below is my pet peeve list of tried-and-true reactivity nightmares. I want you to understand that the reason I get so worked up about these foods is that people are making a concerted effort to include them in their daily diets, and these foods could be triggering everything that is problematic to your health. So all of these foods make me sigh and say they are the devil!

- **Oatmeal.** This is one of those foods that has a reputation for being a superfood but is actually anything but. I can't tell you how many of my clients have eaten oatmeal (which is 85 percent reactive) for years, thinking it's good for them, and have been negatively impacting their health and weight because of its high inflammatory effect! Remember, *inflammation is the underlying factor behind all disease and health issues.* Oatmeal is said to lower cholesterol, and if it's a friendly food for you, then there's a great chance that it might. But if oatmeal is inflammatory for you, there is a great chance that it will actually raise your cholesterol. Remember, inflammation triggers whatever is chronic or latent in your system—including high cholesterol.

- **Salmon.** Salmon seems to make every superfood and anti-inflammatory list, so people are eating it religiously, believing it's doing their bodies good. But we have found salmon to have a whopping 85 percent reactivity rate. Salmon is a fish rich in oils. As soon as you cook fish oil, you start to change its structure, potentially making it inflammatory. Salmon is also rich in omega-3s, which are very unstable when heated; proteins can easily be denatured. When you combine all these potential problems with the fact that salmon can be high in heavy metals, PCBs, and mercury, you can easily see how this "healthy" food could be a potential nightmare.

- **Asparagus.** Asparagus is consistently reactive for the vast majority of our clients. I ask people to limit their test to four or five stalks, as even that much can often cause a one-pound weight gain. It kills me to think of all those people eating tons of asparagus and struggling to lose weight.

- **Tomato sauce.** Any tomato product, like ketchup, salsa, and tomato soup, goes on this list. Tomatoes are naturally high in acid. They fall into the nightshade vegetable family, which is renowned for instigating an inflammatory response. Most canned or bottled tomato products contain citric acid, which further increases the acidity and exacerbates arthritis, psoriasis, eczema, and acid reflux.

- **Tofu.** You already know my feelings on soy, but just to drive the point home: soy interferes with estrogen levels and deactivates the thyroid. In addition, it interferes with zinc absorption; zinc is a staple for immune function as well as prostate and digestive health.

(continued)

- **Black beans.** Chickpeas are low reactive, but black beans, which dieters seem to love, are a whopping 85 percent reactive. Anything that causes gas is a signal that the body is having a hard time digesting that food, and black beans are notorious for this. As we age, we lose digestive enzymes that break down food for digestion and absorption, so those handy "diet" foods like beans that worked so well for us in our twenties will have a very different effect in our forties and beyond.
- **Turkey.** Turkey is 85 percent reactive, so ordering that turkey burger instead of a beef or lamb burger is not likely to help your waistline or your health. How many people eat turkey sandwiches for lunch, thinking it's a healthy option? And don't even get me started on turkey chili…turkey, beans, and tomato paste all in one dish. Thanksgiving dinner? I'm sorry, but you shouldn't get tired after eating something! That's a pretty good indicator that it's having a negative effect on the body.

Understanding Your Chemistry

Very often, my clients experience such astonishing results from the cleanse—in terms of both health benefits and weight loss—that they don't want to leave home, so to speak. People get on a high from how good they're feeling and the weight they're dropping, and they're afraid of trying anything new. But I encourage you not to stop there. Anyone can lose weight for a short time by sticking to just the least reactive foods. But you'll get mind-numbingly bored with eating the same foods over and over, and your inner three-year-old will throw a tantrum. Your body will stop responding to the same stimulus, and you won't learn anything new that will help you in the long run. In fact you may start to develop food sensitivities if you don't rotate your friendly foods. I don't want to tell you long-term what to eat and what not to eat—I want to teach you how to determine for yourself what works for your own body, so you're empowered to make choices on your own. As one client said, "I love that you don't tell us what to eat—you make us figure it out!"

Frustrations can come up when we start testing because all of a sudden, your fabulous losing streak might get interrupted—or in some cases, reversed. But don't panic; you're better equipped for this than you think. If you test reactive to a food, it's helpful to keep a few things in mind:

- Having a reactive response to a food may at first feel frustrating, but the important thing to focus on is that you've rooted out one of your trigger foods—and that's major progress. Once you identify a trigger food, *you never have to eat that food again*. That's your takeaway from this. This is the last time this food will mysteriously sabotage your health or weight. From now on, you'll be in charge.

- Reactivity passes. 24–48 hours is the norm until you get back to the weight you were before the reactive food or the corresponding health symptoms go away, but if you're in a constant state of ill health, it might be closer to 72 hours. In that case, you'll want to repeat two friendly days to allow your body to heal.

- By now, you already have a few friendly days in your arsenal that you can return to whenever you want to lose weight, and by Day Eight, you'll have a solid four to five. Think about that. How long has it been since you've been able to say unequivocally, "Following these days' menus will enable me to feel good and lose weight." Probably quite some time! But now you know how to restore your body's natural homeostasis. Every time you put your body on the path to health, it responds, because it wants to be there.

- Remember: *the number on the scale is nothing more than data*. We're gauging your chemical reaction to foods, and this information is going to help you for the rest of your life. There is no such thing as inexplicable weight gain on The Plan, and I think that's of great comfort. Every day is a chance to learn something new about our bodies. Remember, there are no mistakes, only lessons that we can use for future success. You can always tweak the variables once you pinpoint what didn't work for you. By the end of your twenty days, you will be well on your way to your goal weight (if not at it) and will have a map in hand that shows you how to get there and stay there.

Marco, 48

I had just beat chronic Lyme disease and was going back to the gym since I had packed on an extra 35 pounds throughout my fight with Lyme. In addition, my doctor wanted to put me on a statin to lower my cholesterol. I thought I was eating well, but little did I know that a lot of the foods I thought were good for me were actually working against me, because they were inflammatory. Going to the gym only allowed me to lose 10 lbs., but with The Plan, I was able to easily achieve my goal weight, and drop my cholesterol to a level not requiring any medication, in three weeks!

Reading Your Body's Signals

You already know the signs to look for in terms of reactivity. Weight gain, increase in or new appearance of chronic or latent health issues (this can run the gamut from skin flare-ups to joint pain and more), digestive disturbances (gas, constipation, etc.), depression or extreme emotionality, insomnia, hormonal imbalance, and fatigue are some of the signals that our chemistry is not reacting well. You shouldn't suddenly get a headache after a meal...or be tired...or look in the mirror and notice bags under your eyes that weren't there a few hours earlier. One of my clients told me that she tested pork and it made her feel bloated and sleepy, and she wanted to know if that meant she was reactive. Yes, 100 percent! Anything that makes you sick, causes pain, or makes you feel just plain "off" in any way is triggering a reactive response. Once you put your body on the path to health, it does not want to get off and it will send you a myriad of signs. You'll start to be able to spot these bodily responses very quickly. Soon you won't need me, because you'll be learning all the ways besides weight that your body is constantly talking to you.

The Plan is structured so that you should lose roughly half a pound per day until you reach your set point and feel *great*. When you lose less than that, gain, or experience any negative health responses on The Plan, it is always for one of the four reasons listed below. At the heart of The Plan is learning how to become your own body whisperer. I'm going to help you do the detective work so you can easily pinpoint what's caused the response and make informed choices going forward.

Michelle, 66

Since my late twenties, I've experienced debilitating headaches that could last up to ten days. Despite explorations down both traditional and nontraditional paths, the headaches have persisted. I have been to the finest ENT doctors, neurologists, headache specialists, TMJ specialists, allergists, and more. I've tried homeopathic treatments, acupuncture, naturopathy, and massage, and have seen every kind of healer. I do use medications if desperately needed, but the side effects of those are often worse than the headache! Despite trying literally just about everything, I kept looking for healers out there who might be able to help or at least allay some of the symptoms and pain.

I read an article about Lyn-Genet and noticed that many of the comments were from people who suffered from headaches and whose symptoms lessened with her guidance. I sensed there could be something in her work that could contribute to unlocking a door toward healing. I made the call.

While I consider myself someone with a good foundation and understanding about food and a basic understanding of how different things "challenge" your body, Lyn-Genet's fact-based and intuitive insight into physical issues was stunning.

(continued)

A simple example: among my favorite foods are (were) aged balsamic vinegar, as well as arugula and strawberries. Under Lyn-Genet's food direction and by keeping a food log, headache log, and basal body temperature log, I discovered that these foods and some others were "drivers" in my headaches because of thyroid issues. Who would ever have imagined that to be the case? I found Lyn-Genet's unique combination of knowledge about food and its properties and how it interacts in one's body immensely useful.

I would honestly say that after working with Lyn-Genet my headache symptoms have absolutely declined. And while they are not gone completely, I can usually point to the series of circumstances that might prompt a big headache, and that is part of the influence of her work.

With headaches, people look at you askance (is it stress, are you crazy?) or just prescribe medication. That is not the case here. It required vigilance, and in my experience, it was well worth it. For me, The Plan remains a great experience that continues to pay off!

Reasons for Reactivity

- **You didn't meet your water intake requirements or drank water after dinner.** This is always the first place to look. For every sixteen ounces less than your required amount that you drink, the body will hold on to half a pound. Dehydration also exacerbates an inflammatory response, so even if you had a very mild reaction to a food, it can become a full-blown one. Overdrinking and drinking after dinner almost always shows up on the scale as water weight. Does that mean you'll never again be able to drink water after dinner? No. But it's best to avoid doing so during the testing phase, when we are trying to precisely identify which foods do and don't work for you—you don't want to throw in another variable. If you feel like you're constantly thirsty, this means hydration is not getting to the tissues properly. We find that adding some lemon juice to your water during the day takes care of that nicely, as it makes the water more alkaline and the Vitamin C increases hydration levels.

- **You've had too much sodium.** Sodium exacerbates inflammation and causes water retention as well. We have The Plan structured to keep your daily sodium intake to the American Heart Association's recommended daily amount of 1,500 milligrams. If you've followed the menu plan and added only a moderate amount of sea salt, this shouldn't be an issue. Excess sodium generally shows up as a problem when you're dining out, since restaurants hide so much salt in their food—regardless of whether you are eating at high-end restaurants, diners, or fast-food establishments. So if you've dined out and stuck to your friendly foods only and gained weight, you'll know that the restaurant used too much salt and that you may not want to eat there again. Why should you pay to gain weight?
- **You overexercised.** We'll go into more detail about the guidelines for exercise on The Plan, but for now, the rule of thumb is that exercising more than four times a week or doing extreme workouts can create a state of inflammation in the body that is counterproductive and stunts weight loss—or even causes weight gain.
- **You've eaten a food that is reactive for you.** If you've ruled out the possible causes above, then you know for certain that a food you've eaten is reactive for you. You'll know precisely which one it is because we introduce only one new test food each testing day. If you've had your water and stuck to the sodium requirements and exercise guidelines, you've got your answer.

If you find you are reactive to a food, you'll want to do the following day as a "rest day," to give your body a chance to recover. A rest day is any day that has thus far proven friendly for you. When the body is in an inflamed state, it's difficult to get an accurate reading if you're then immediately testing something new. You want to give your body a chance to repair. When you start to connect the dots and see how looking after your health first always results in weight loss, you will create a much healthier relationship to food. You'll see as you proceed through Days Six through Twenty that we have built-in rest days between tests.

Putting Your Data to Work for You

It's important to remember that just because you test reactive to a food, that doesn't mean you can't have it ever again. If the inflammatory response was moderate (up to a half-pound weight gain with no accompanying physiological response), then going forward, you might want to incorporate that food only occasionally, say once every seven to ten days. Just make sure to follow that day with a friendly day to allow the body to repair any inflammation. It is when we have inflammatory day after inflammatory day that we start to see eroding health and weight gain.

If the reactive response is more extreme, in terms of either weight gain or physical symptoms, I recommend avoiding that food for right now and retesting it in three to six months. Omitting a reactive food will decrease inflammation, and your body will heal. Sometimes that means it can once again do great on a food that tested reactive for you the first time around. (This is why your blood work can show different results every time you test for allergies and sensitivities.) Keep using your scale as your gauge to determine your body's response. It's important to note that you will most likely always have a sensitivity to this food, so keep applying your data of weight gain/loss/stabilization to determine how often you should eat this food. (The general guidelines I recommend are no more than twice a month, but you can play around with what works best for you.)

If a food has an extreme reactive effect on you, then it would make sense to avoid it altogether. Inflammation is cumulative, and when you repeatedly trigger it, your health and weight issues increase exponentially. Current digestive problems like bloating or gas can turn into IBS; a small weight increase escalates into a big one; moderately high cholesterol turns into severely high cholesterol—and a risk to your heart health. To me, it's a clear choice: why in the world would you want to continue eating a food that is making you sick and overweight?

The good news is that once your body recognizes a reactive food, you tend not to want it anymore. When you are eating healthfully, your palate changes. I know that might sound implausible to you right now, but I've seen this play out again and again. One couple in their late thirties whom I worked with, Ken and Jenny, sailed through their Plan. When their twenty days were over, they went out to celebrate at their favorite pizza spot. They took one bite and promptly walked out of the pizza place because it just didn't taste good anymore. Helena, age forty-two, loved omelets, so she tested eggs. Her weight was up .6 pounds the next day. What was interesting was that she told me that while she was eating the eggs, the smell was slightly repulsive to her—which had never happened before. When things like that happen, it's a sign from the body—listen to it! The point here is that you may not need to worry about working in your favorite food after all. Your body may very naturally take care of your cravings for the better as you lead it along the path to health.

Exercise and The Plan

Karen, thirty-two, worked out like crazy, trying to lose fifteen pounds. Her husband was a trainer and had convinced her that to lose weight, you needed to exercise more and count calories to ensure an optimal calorie in/calorie out ratio. The formula wasn't working, and Karen's weight continued to build slowly year after year. To add to that, she started getting frequent headaches—and she was trying to get pregnant. Overall, it was a pretty frustrating time for her.

Karen came to me for help. We cut her workouts down to three or four times a week and started her on The Plan. Within a month, she'd lost twelve pounds and her constant headaches had vanished. Even better, three months later, she was pregnant!

Like Karen, many people believe that exercising more causes greater weight loss. We believe that because it's what we've always been told by fitness experts. But the science of our body chemistry proves otherwise. Overexercising puts your body through stress. If you're exercising day after day, your body gets the message that it needs to hold on to more calories to keep up with the energetic demands. It doesn't know how much energy it will need, so it adapts to the energy requirements you are programming into it and holds on to more and more calories for potential future survival. This is why chronic exercisers have trouble losing weight.

Please don't get me wrong: I am a huge proponent of exercise when it's done right and reasonably. It's important for so many reasons: cardiovascular health, stress reduction, mood elevation, bone density, and a sense of well-being and confidence, to name just a few.

The key words here are *when it's done right and reasonably.* If you are working out for stress relief, that's great—and smart. But if you're exercising intensely to lose weight, it's probably not going to work. The body burns the most energy when it's doing repair, not when it's exercising. If you look at the caloric expenditure when you're exercising, it can be nominal. But when you're sleeping and doing deep repair, you can lose two pounds! Body builders and athletes know you need periods of rest if you want to promote muscle growth.

We recommend exercising no more than four times per week. We have found that people who consistently exercise six days a week lose weight 25 percent more slowly than people who exercise four days a week. In addition, their health conditions do not improve as rapidly! It would be a shame to put so much effort into your diet trying to be healthy and sabotage it because you're exercising too much.

Finding what exercise works best for your body and the optimal frequency, intensity, and duration is really important. Exercise types and duration can be tested, just like foods. You take any friendly day and you replicate it, inserting exercise as the variable. We'll cover this in more detail in Part Three and in the Five-Day Self-Test in Part Five. But for now, until you can test, I recommend either thirty minutes of cardio no more than four times per week or light weight training for the same amount of time, and yoga that is not heated.

If Weight Loss Is Slow to Kick In

When you have "beaten up" your body through overexercise (also known as overtraining) and severe calorie deprivation, it will hold on to weight as a defense mechanism. Its goal is to keep you alive, and when you program it to think that it always needs a reserve to live off, it's going to hold on to your fat for dear life. If you've been living on deprivation diets and overtraining, it may take your body a while to realize that you've slowed down and that adequate nutrients and calories are coming in on a regular basis. When your body starts to realize that it no longer needs to guard against unhealthy stimulus—which it will very soon if you stick with The Plan—it will respond with appropriate weight loss.

Some people stabilize every two to three days, and then all of a sudden, the body lets go of weight. If you find yourself in this category, you might wonder how long it will take for you to lose weight normally. We find that within two to three weeks of following The Plan and doing moderate exercise, the body realizes that the "attack" is over, and the weight starts to fly off. If you'd like, at that point, you can always redo your plan from Day Two onward to gather updated data on how your body reacts to the test foods.

Lauryn, 44

When I began The Plan with Lyn-Genet, I was working out four to five hours per week and had eliminated dairy, wine, beer, meat, and poultry, with the once-a-week indulgence in fish and an egg.

(continued)

I was fighting to just maintain my weight and was losing that battle as my weight began to creep up again. I blamed my hypothyroidism. However, I was determined to win the Battle of the Bulge and every day I was battling hard like a warrior! Working out, researching weight loss, making healthy choices, but never confident they were healthy for me because they were not yielding the results that were promised, and then giving up because I wasn't getting results. I was hungry, I was tired, I was emotional, and I was gaining.

Yet not one person I knew who had tried The Plan was failing. They were eating so many calories and they had hypothyroidism, other health issues, etc. They were having insane success—and it was fast! For me, one to two pounds a month was the best I could do on my own if I stayed at 1,200 calories a day. And I was hungry—all the time. I figured that if this was what things were like at age forty for me, then by age fifty, I would only be able to eat rice and water and need to work out two hours a day just to maintain. That sounded miserable! I wanted to live life, but I also wanted to be healthy and have the energy to enjoy it—to travel—even just to stay awake for it!

In come Lyn-Genet and The Plan: I lost 3.2 pounds in the first three days, and about twenty days after that, I had reached my goal weight. Best of all, I am keeping it off and enjoying food. I never count calories and I love finishing my day with wine and chocolate. The food is absolutely delicious!

I work out zero to two hours a week now and have so much more time to do the things I love as a result. I have energy! I used to *need* my morning cup of coffee, but now it is optional (and I don't get a caffeine headache when I skip it). PMS used to hijack two weeks out of my month, which is at least six months out of the year (so wrong!). I used to get miserable emotional swings and appetite fluctuations during that time; now I am just even keel throughout with no bloating or weight gain. I *love* that.

The bottom line: I needed someone to teach me how to eat to finally change all this. I will be forever grateful to Lyn and The Plan.

The Daily Basics of the Testing Phase

Just as you did during the cleanse, every morning upon awakening you'll record your weight and take your liver detox supplement or tonic. Your daily water intake is still calculated according to your weight and activity levels, and the general guidelines for the daily menus stay the same:

- Follow as closely as possible the set menu plans without deviating, eliminating, or substituting anything. Remember, the days are all chemically structured!
- Stick to eating at meals and snack times only. If you're hungry in between, there's a good chance you're dehydrated, so remember to drink your water.
- Eat until you are full at breakfast, lunch, and dinner.

For optimum success, eat your meals at home for as many days as possible. Dining out is a test that we do on Day Eighteen. You want to test a restaurant by ordering your friendly foods (you don't want to test a new food at a restaurant, because the sodium variable can throw off your data), so I want you to have as many friendly foods as possible under your belt before venturing out!

If it's not possible for you to eat at home for seventeen days—and I fully appreciate that it might not be—you can feel free to move Day Eighteen to any other day in your rotation. In other words, if on Day Nine you know you have a dinner plan at a restaurant, substitute Day Eighteen's menu plan for Day Nine's. You will have to have enough knowledge of which foods work with your chemistry, as you want to stick to ordering your friendly foods when dining out. If you "pass" the restaurant test, then you can pick up where you left off the following day. If you are retaining too much water from the sodium, take a rest day, and then you can resume. Everything you need to know about how to test a restaurant is listed on page 142, under "The Inside Scoop on Day Eighteen." One caveat: this switching of days only applies to Day Eighteen; all the others are truly best done in their proper order.

If any questions come up for you during the testing phase, you can go to www.lyngenet.com for more information, as well as helpful tips, ideas, and stories from other Plan followers to help you along the way.

Please note that the menu listed here is the Winter Menu, meant for colder times of the year. We have seasonal menus because the body responds differently to different foods according to temperature. For the Spring Menu, meant for warmer times of the year, please see Part Five. If you live in a warm climate year-round, then by all means you can go straight to the Spring Menu. Your clothing should be the gauge: whenever (or wherever) you can consistently dress in just one layer, the Spring Menu is the way to go.

Note: You can download updated days 1–20 at www.lyngenet.com.

Katherine, 53

While I was someone who had exercised her whole adult life and maintained her weight even through three pregnancies, I found myself at fifty-two with eight pounds that had simply settled around my middle, creating serious muffin top!

I had borderline high blood pressure and cholesterol and was chronically constipated. I was dismayed and frustrated. Nothing seemed to work anymore. In full-blown menopause, I thought this was simply what happens to women as they age.

What The Plan did for me was change my relationship with food. Since I have a very stressful job as a wedding designer, I relied on food to deal with the stress. For the most part, I was eating foods that I thought were healthy but for me really weren't. I was so unaware of how much salt and sugar is in the average diet. Even the "healthy" supplements that I was taking were not meeting my needs.

I must admit the first few days on The Plan were hard, but what soon came over me was startling. I felt so good, happy and energetic—life was great! I was hooked. This was the feeling that I needed to work well in my job.

Eating this way made a difference in my life in so many ways. I dropped my eight pounds, and the very best part was that my blood pressure decreased and my cholesterol dropped twenty-five points in only twenty days! Yes, I do indulge in pizza and beer on occasion, but it is a treat and not a need. I no longer look for food to get me through my life or use it as a reward. Besides, on The Plan I can have chocolate and red wine every day and cream in my coffee without guilt! Through The Plan I have learned what works best for me.

Day Four: Cheese

If coffee, chocolate, and wine were a part of your life, as of today they are happily back in your repertoire. And on Day Four we test one of life's greatest pleasures, as far as I'm concerned: cheese.

UPON AWAKENING

- Weigh yourself and record the results in your Plan Journal.
- Drink 16 ounces of fresh water with lemon juice (after you weigh yourself).
- Take your liver support supplement and/or drink a cup of dandelion tea.

BREAKFAST

For women: 1 cup of flax granola with ½ cup of blueberries,
½ apple, or ½ pear
For men: 1½ cups of flax granola with 1 cup of blueberries or
1 whole apple or pear
Silk coconut milk or Rice Dream

LUNCH

Leftover Roasted Italian Winter Vegetables (1 cup for women, 2 to
3 cups for men) on a bed of spinach with pumpkin seeds and
1 ounce of goat cheese

SNACK

Carrots with up to 6 tablespoons of Homemade Hummus (page
181) or raw almond butter (1 to 2 tablespoons for women, 3
to 4 tablespoons for men) or a ½ piece of fruit (full piece for
men) with sunflower seeds

Why Homemade Hummus?

Store-bought or restaurant hummus can be up to 90 percent reactive
for people over forty years old. It contains tahini, made from sesame
seeds, which is high in omega-6. Omega-6 is the pro-inflammatory
omega oil and the sesame oil goes rancid quickly. Research shows
that sesame seed allergies are on the rise; in some countries such as
Australia, sesame seeds rank right after milk, eggs, and peanuts. The
Plan's Homemade Hummus recipe is easy to make, tastes every bit as
good as, if not better than, commercial kinds, and ensures that you
won't trigger an inflammatory response.

DINNER

Chicken with Mango Salsa (page 176)

Arugula with carrots and ¼ avocado (make enough to have some
left over for lunch on Day Five)

Steamed or sautéed broccoli and onions with Orange Oil
(page 176) and chili flakes

DESSERT

1 ounce of dark chocolate or Cinnamon Poached Fruit (page 185)
with optional Katie's Whipped Coconut Cream (page 296)

WATER

Be sure to drink your recommended daily water intake throughout the day, ending by dinner.

The Inside Scoop on Day Four

Here's everything you might want to know about Day Four's new foods:

Coffee

For all you coffee lovers: enjoy!

A cup of coffee in the morning can be very emotionally satisfying. I do find, however, that any coffee not drunk as morning coffee can show up as weight gain, so it's best for The Plan's purposes to stick to a cup just in the morning. Avoid decaf if you can and go for darker-roast coffee, like French Roast, which has less acid.

If you would like to add sugar to your coffee, that's perfectly fine. Same with agave nectar and honey. Please continue to avoid artificial sweeteners, however; they are highly toxic, impede weight loss, and damage your health. My experience with clients has shown that Stevia also impedes weight loss, so best to avoid that as well.

For now, until we test milk (which is highly reactive), please stick to either Silk coconut creamer, rice milk, or half-and-half. Why half-and-half over milk? Because the reactive and allergenic potential of milk comes from the milk sugars and proteins, and fat buffers the sugar absorption. The more fat a milk product contains, the less these substances can affect our health and weight. Heavy cream would be even less reactive. Ideally, you always want to have fat along with sugar, to mitigate the glycemic rush. Skim and low-fat milk are harder to digest and actually hinder weight loss; removing the fat leads to sugar spikes, which eventually leads to weight gain. In fact, low-fat dairy products have been linked to the rise in type 2 diabetes.

Plus, because the brain is 60 percent fat and our cell walls have a phospholipid barrier (which is composed of fatty acids), we want to make sure to get enough fat in our diet for brain function and immune enhancement. That doesn't mean having heavy whipped cream all day—we want healthy fats like olive oil, avocado, nuts, and seeds—but using half-and-half is a good start to the day, and the fat will also buffer the acidity of the coffee.

Cheese

Milk, yogurt, and cheese all test differently in terms of reactivity. We start with cheese because it is the least reactive—and goat cheese is less reactive than cow's cheese, which is why we test that first. Many people think goat cheese is just the soft, white kind, but just about any cheese you like as a cow's cheese you can now get as goat cheese. Goat Cheddar and goat Gouda are delicious and widely available. I'm telling you, even your kids will like goat Cheddar; they'll never know the difference!

Wine

Ah, wine!

A glass of wine is a wonderful way to wind down and relax. Red wine, which is what we include on The Plan (white wine is more acidic, so for right now we'll avoid it; remember, you can always test it later), has terrific health and weight loss benefits. At the end of a long day, many people can feel wound up and tense, which hampers digestion. Stress is a big factor in our society, and the stress hormone cortisol is notorious for impeding weight loss. Wine decreases our stress, and in turn, that lowers cortisol. When our systems are at ease, we digest better; and when we ease digestion, we lose more weight. Wine is also a diuretic that helps flush excess water from our system. And according to a study published in the *American Journal of Clinical Nutrition*, red wine may even benefit digestive health—much like a probiotic—by improving the balance of good bacteria in the gut. It has also been proven to kill bacteria such as E coli, salmonella, *Staphylococcus aureus,* and *Klebsiella pneumoniae.* When you put all those things together, you're going to get good results.

I've had people say that they love wine, but they want to lose more weight so they skip it while on The Plan. But that, my friend, is a mistake! Repeatedly I've seen wine enhance clients' weight loss once they start to include it. Certainly if you're dining out, you're going to benefit from having a glass, because its diuretic effects will counteract any excess sodium in the restaurant food and the potential weight gain you might see as a result.

Even beyond the physical benefits, wine is a great joy. Happiness offsets inflammation. Seriously. I'm not kidding. The whole philosophy of The Plan is that you can lose weight in a joyful manner. Wine is a very pleasurable part of our culture that encourages us to slow down, linger at the end of a meal (which of course aids digestion), and enjoy good company and happy times. On The Plan, you are creating a lifelong blueprint for your lifestyle and way of eating, and as far as I'm concerned, relishing the good things in life should be a significant part of that.

Chocolate

Speaking of the good things in life…

I love how happy people get when I tell them they can enjoy dark chocolate—*every day*! We start with an ounce, and then later you can test larger portions. The interesting thing is that when you can have chocolate daily, you don't feel the need to overindulge. My only qualifier is to please make sure that it is 65 percent cacao or less. Higher than that and the chocolate gets too acidic; this can trigger inflammation and acid reflux. If you want to have chocolate with nuts in it, please stick to almonds until you have tested other nuts later on.

Keeping an Eye on Yeast

If you reintroduced wine, chocolate, or vinegar today, be sure to check your tongue tomorrow morning to see if there is any yeast reaction. A white coating indicates that there's a yeast overgrowth, which you can remedy with probiotics. The use of MSM also enhances the efficacy of probiotics. If you do experience a yeast reaction, please avoid vinegar and wine *or* chocolate for a week, until you can retest (no cutting out both wine *and* chocolate…we don't scale back on joy that way!).

Day Five: Rye

On Day Five we introduce rye. We test rye as the first grain (besides rice) because it is very similar in its structure to wheat, but it contains a prebiotic, which aids in digestion.

Rye crackers, which are what we test, are much lower in sodium and yeast than bread—plus they have a very satisfying crunch. People often ask what kind of rye cracker to get. We find that the light rye is enjoyed by most, and we have not noticed any difference in reactivity between different brands.

UPON AWAKENING

- Weigh yourself and record the results in your Plan Journal.
- Drink 16 ounces of fresh water with lemon juice (after you weigh yourself).
- Take your liver support supplement and/or drink a cup of dandelion tea.

BREAKFAST

For women: 1 cup flax granola with ½ cup of blueberries,
½ apple, or ½ pear

For men: 1½ cups flax granola with 1 cup of blueberries or
1 whole apple or pear

Silk coconut milk or Rice Dream

LUNCH

Leftover dinner salad from Day Four with added goat cheese

Cream of Broccoli Soup (page 294)

SNACK

For women: 1 rye cracker with 1 to 2 tablespoons of raw almond
butter and ½ apple

For men: 2 rye crackers with 3 to 4 tablespoons of raw almond
butter and 1 whole apple

DINNER

Chicken with Spicy Apricot Glaze (page 177) on a bed of arugula
Sautéed zucchini with onion and basil topped with Orange Oil
(page 176) and 2 tablespoons grated Manchego (make enough
to have some left over for lunch on Day Six)
Beet and Carrot Salad (page 178) with sunflower seeds

DESSERT

1 ounce of dark chocolate or Cinnamon Poached Fruit (page 185)
with optional Katie's Whipped Coconut Cream (page 296)

WATER

Be sure to drink your recommended daily water intake throughout the day, ending by dinner.

The Inside Scoop on Day Five

Rye is a pivotal test, because it will help inform us how your body
may tolerate wheat, and knowing your sensitivity to wheat is very
important. For The Plan's purposes, rye is a "gateway" grain. If you
do well on rye, it doesn't necessarily guarantee that bread and other
grains will be friendly for you, but it does increase the odds.

If You Test Reactive for Rye

Don't despair...this does not mean that all crackers and breads are
out of the question for you. You can still test bread made from wheat
on Day Eight; there is just a slightly higher chance that it might not
work. You can also repeat Day Five anytime and just choose any alternate cracker you like. Rice is easily processed for many people, so you
can always try rice crackers and rice bread. In six months, you can test
problematic grains again. The overall state of decreased inflammation
in your body from being on The Plan may mean that the next time
around, rye will process as friendlier for you.

Day Six: Protein

Day Six is the first protein test. Right now you have chicken and several vegetarian sources of protein in your friendly arsenal, but the body adapts to repeated stimulus, so it's important to add a few more. You want to keep rotating your proteins for weight loss and health benefits. Some people get into a friendly-foods groove that can quickly turn into a rut because they are afraid to test new proteins. The body responds to foods you eat repeatedly just the way it does to exercise: you need to keep altering the stimulus to avoid a plateau and potential food sensitivities. Then you'll continue to get the results you're looking for.

We first test the friendliest animal proteins, which are listed below.

UPON AWAKENING

- Weigh yourself and record the results in your Plan Journal.
- Drink 16 ounces of fresh water with lemon juice (after you weigh yourself).
- Take your liver support supplement and/or drink a cup of dandelion tea.

BREAKFAST

For women: 1 cup of flax granola with choice of approved fruit (½ cup of blueberries, ½ apple, or ½ pear)

For men: 1½ cups of flax granola with choice of approved fruit (1 cup of blueberries or 1 whole apple or pear)

Silk coconut milk or Rice Dream

LUNCH

Baby romaine with leftover sautéed zucchini and goat cheese

Cream of Broccoli Soup (page 294) or Steamed Broccoli with EVO

For women: 1 rye cracker with 1 to 2 tablespoons of raw almond butter

For men: 2 rye crackers with 3 to 4 tablespoons of raw almond butter

SNACK

> For women: ½ piece of approved fruit and a small handful of raw
> almonds
> For men: 1 whole piece of fruit and a small handful of raw
> almonds

DINNER

> Choose your protein to test on a bed of mixed greens:
> Wild white fish
> Steak
> Lamb
> Venison
> Duck
> Egg
> Roasted Squash, Kale, and Manchego Salad (page 179) (make

enough to have some left over for lunch on Day Seven)

DESSERT

> 1 ounce of dark chocolate or Cinnamon Poached Fruit (page 185)
> with optional Katie's Whipped Coconut Cream (page 296)

WATER

> Be sure to drink your recommended daily water intake through-
> out the day, ending by dinner.

The Inside Scoop on Day Six

Here is what you might want to know about some of the proteins you
might be choosing to test today:

Beef

Beef is often vilified, but we have actually found it to be very
friendly—lower reactive, even, than fish! The trick is to know how
often you should eat it. Beef can be a little tough on digestion, so most

people do well if they have beef only once every seven days or so. If you do choose to test beef as your first protein, make sure you love chicken as well, because for now those will be your two main animal proteins, and chicken will have to fill in on the days in between.

People often ask if different cuts of beef react differently. We haven't found that much of a difference, so choose whichever one you like best. Flank steak is usually marinated, however, so be sure to watch out for that extra sodium. Personally, I like the fattier cuts of beef because they're so much more flavorful.

It's best to cook your steak medium-rare. Remember, fats in proteins are unstable, and the longer you cook them, the more reactive they become. So if you like your steak well done, you'd be better off with a leaner cut like filet mignon. Beef carpaccio—which isn't cooked at all—burns the cleanest and is a terrific option to choose if you're dining out.

Lamb

Many people are afraid of lamb because they say it tastes gamy, but you'd be hard pressed to taste the difference between a hamburger and a good lamb burger (we've found that ground lamb tests the best of all the lamb varieties). And unlike beef, you can eat lamb up to three times a week.

The big difference between the two is that lamb is easier to digest. So if you love denser proteins, lamb burgers might be the way to go. The recipe for Lamb Burgers on page 184 is a major favorite. In fact, the first time one mom on The Plan made them, her whole family couldn't get enough of them... including her normally vegan husband!

Fish

I find that most people over forty have an uneasy truce with fish. It is 40 percent or more reactive, depending on the type of fish, and when it's consumed more than once or twice a week, it often causes weight stabilization. I have many clients who are pescatarians and have a hard time losing weight if they don't factor in other sources of protein.

To give your body the best chance of responding well to fish, we test first on wild white fish. Farm-raised fish are rife with toxic substances. Extensive analysis has been done on farm-raised fish, showing that they contain high concentrations of contaminants widely known to be carcinogenic. They also can contain high levels of mercury and aquaculture chemicals that are absorbed into the tissue of the fish (antibiotics, pesticides, antiparasitic drugs, hormones, etc.), which we then ingest. Our bodies will recognize these chemicals as toxic invaders and trigger an inflammatory response to fight them off.

You can choose halibut, sole, haddock...almost any white fish, as long as it's wild. For now, please avoid tuna, cod, and swordfish; those can be tested later on.

Eggs

Eggs are almost on par with fish in terms of reactivity potential, but unlike fish, they are fine to consume every other day. Daily use is a much harder test. You can try something simple like an omelet or fried, poached, or scrambled eggs—anything other than hard-boiled. Raising the temperature of eggs that much denatures the protein, which causes greater potential for reactivity.

Venison

Wild game, such as venison and bison, is fantastic and lower reactive than many of the more problematic proteins. It's interesting to note, however, that because it is so much higher in omega-3s, overcooking it can definitely turn this friendly food into a reactive one. So venison stew might not be the best first test. Instead, opt for the venison carpaccio or tenderloin cooked rare to medium.

Duck

While it may not be the easiest thing to source for some, duck breast is worth the search. Duck is as low reactive as chicken, so it will be an easy second protein to add to your list of friendly foods. Plus, in

Chinese medicine, duck is known for helping edema and many hormonal problems.

Duck breast is easy to prepare because it's just like chicken. Most people like it best cooked medium rare (my favorite). All you need to do is marinate in your choice of sauces from the list of recipes in Part Four, pan-sear it with its own fat for flavor, then remove the fat and enjoy!

Beans

Beans are not low reactive, but I include them as an option on Day Six for anyone who would prefer to incorporate another vegetarian protein rather than animal. Many vegetarian sources of protein do seem to be harder to digest for people over the age of thirty-five. That being said, we have worked with many vegetarians and vegans and were successful in finding what works for them.

The interesting thing about beans that most people don't realize is that you don't have to group beans and rice in the same meal to make a complete protein—which is best for The Plans purposes, since that is a potentially problematic pairing. You have twenty-four to thirty-six hours for them to combine into a complete protein, which increases your odds of success for health and weight loss.

I recommend starting with lentils or pinto beans. Please avoid black beans for now, as they are highly reactive.

Jordyn, 36

To be completely honest, I'd never stuck with any type of food plan longer than three days. I'm currently on Day Seven of The Plan and going strong. I'm sure it's a combination of factors: it's tailored to me, it's healing my body, I'm full after every meal, and it produces results. I've learned so much about myself in the past seven days. I never realized how much I used food as a crutch. I'm learning to deal with my days and my emotions differently now. It hasn't been easy, but it is oh so *very* worth it.

Day Seven: Rest Day

After a few days on The Plan, we take a one-day break from testing. From here on, as the reactivity levels of foods may increase, every other day will be a rest day to allow your body to reset.

UPON AWAKENING

- Weigh yourself and record the results in your Plan Journal.
- Drink 16 ounces of fresh water with lemon juice (after you weigh yourself).
- Take your liver support supplement and/or drink a cup of dandelion tea.

BREAKFAST

For women: 1 cup of flax granola with choice of approved fruit
For men: 1½ cups of flax granola with choice of approved fruit
Silk coconut milk or Rice Dream

LUNCH

Leftover Roasted Squash, Kale, and Manchego Salad with pumpkin seeds (reheat)
½ an apple for women; whole apple for men

The Powerful Pumpkin Seed

Pumpkin seeds pack 9 grams of protein into a single ounce; are rich in zinc, which is important for your immune system; and are great for prostate health. All of my clients carry pumpkin seeds around with them because they are such an easy, inexpensive way to quickly add protein to a salad or sandwich when you're on the run.

SNACK

1 ounce of salt-free or low sodium (under 70 mg per ounce) potato chips

DINNER

Chicken with Lemon Garlic Sauce (page 175) on a bed of arugula
Sautéed vegetables (Swiss chard, broccoli, carrots, zucchini,
onions, and shiitakes with garlic, herbs of choice, and Orange
Oil (page 176); make enough to have some left over for dinner
on Day Eight)

DESSERT

1 ounce of dark chocolate or Cinnamon Poached Fruit (page 185)
with optional Katie's Whipped Coconut Cream (page 296)

WATER

Be sure to drink your recommended daily water intake throughout the day, ending by dinner.

The Inside Scoop on Day Seven

It's always an option to include a rest day at any point during The
Plan if you feel your body needs it (you'll have several more options
for rest day templates in the days to come). Rest days are ideal when:

- You have a reactive day with physical symptoms. A rest day
  allows the body to heal.
- Your weight is up. A rest day is always a good option to get
  back on track. We never test when weight is up, because that
  signals you are in a state of inflammation and you are more
  likely to test reactively. It's just not kind to the body to pile
  on inflammatory day after inflammatory day; that won't work
  for weight or health. When we are kind to the body, a good
  response follows.
- You know you are going to have a particularly hectic or stressful day. Stress floods your body with cortisol, which interferes
  with weight loss. And stress, of course, negatively impacts your

mental and physical health. Anytime your body is in a compromised state and testing conditions are not optimal, stick with a friendly day.

Until you learn how to construct your own menus in Part Three, please do not deviate from the daily menu plans for rest days (you can always insert any friendly day that has worked for you thus far as a rest day, as long as you follow that full day's menu). The chemical balance ensures proper nutrients and weight loss.

For some clients, seeing potato chips listed as a snack on Day Seven sets off all kinds of dieting alarm bells. We've all been so programmed to believe that we can't have potato chips and lose weight, but on The Plan, it's not only allowed—it's encouraged!

Potatoes are a well-known source of potassium, which is important for weight loss, as it negates sodium. Plus, potatoes are emotionally satisfying. People are shoveling in bananas daily for potassium, but potato chips can easily surpass bananas in potassium content, while bananas contain a huge amount of starch and sugar that cause weight gain.

Or to satisfy their craving for a crunchy treat, many people turn to the supposedly healthy option of microwave popcorn, which is unfortunately carcinogenic. In fact, the renowned Dana-Farber Cancer Institute included microwave popcorn on its list of top 10 foods to avoid because of the toxic chemicals in the linings of the bags, which, when exposed to high heat such as the microwave, can spread into the popcorn. Even air-popped popcorns can be problematic because most are made of genetically modified organisms (GMOs)—and corn is 90 percent reactive. Suddenly potato chips don't seem so scary, do they?

Remember, too, that I'm not suggesting you eat great heaping quantities of potato chips (I'm recommending 1 ounce for women and 1 to 2 ounces for men). *Anything* that you eat too much of isn't good for you. Eat too much broccoli and you'll have gas, which causes digestive issues. What we are trying to establish is a way of eating that is nutrient dense *and* feels like a treat. If you truly don't like potato chips, you can always have half a piece of fruit and nuts or Katie's Kale Chips (page 211). But if you want to loosen some of the restrictions you may have put on yourself in the name of being "healthy," now's the time to do it!

Being on The Plan isn't about being perfect. And it's definitely not about avoiding what you want to eat. We include foods like salt-free potato chips and desserts because people are already consuming these foods. We simply take what people are already eating and wanting and choose a healthier form of it. Let's be realistic and just make better choices, and things will fall into place. I've had so many parents on The Plan say to me that they're so happy to finally be able to keep chips in the house. Their kids love them, and the parents are so much happier that their kids are eating these and not sneaking out and having the highly salted ones elsewhere.

Salt-free chips used to be relegated to health food stores, but you can find them almost anywhere these days. Lay's, Wise, Utz, and other companies have come out with their own versions, available at most supermarkets. Trader Joe's version is my personal favorite.

Weeks Three and Four on The Plan

Admittedly, Days Eight through Fourteen are when I start losing some friends, as we start testing some higher-reactive foods. But it's essential to remember two things: first, the more foods we test, the more friendly ones you will add to your rotation. And second, even if some foods don't work, a lot of foods that you love do—and many others will!

Something magical happens in that third week: people start to realize that if you test reactive to something and gain weight on, say, Day Fourteen, it's really no big deal, because you can just follow with a friendly day on Day Fifteen and the weight comes right back off. You're learning how to plug in and move around variables so you can continue to both test *and* lose weight. It's really that simple.

Day Eight: Bread

People have become carb terrified. But not all carbs are bad—and neither are all breads! Regular bread is less than 20 percent reactive. Before we throw the baby out with the bathwater, so to speak, we're going to test simple bread to see how your body responds.

For this first bread test, please make sure that it is *plain white or wheat bread*. No multigrain, no sprouted-grain, no high-fiber, no bagels. Bagels have a much higher gluten content, and multigrain and sprouted-grain products can have ten or more things in there like oat, corn, millet, lentils, etc. If all those things work for you, great. But every grain is its own test, and odds are you're going to be reactive to at least one or two (corn and oats, for example, are highly reactive). We're going to get a base line on your sensitivity with white or whole wheat and then move on to testing others.

The Multigrain Myth

More isn't necessarily better when it comes to grains or fiber. Remember that your weight is really just your chemical response to food, and if you ingest a multigrain, high-fiber product that contains something you are reactive to, more actually turns out to be a deficit.

One of my all-time classic stories from The Plan was Dan, age fifty-three, who had digestive problems and had been told for years by his doctor that he was gluten intolerant. He'd been living off gluten-free products, but the weight was piling on and his digestion was getting worse. This didn't surprise me at all, since many of these products are made with ingredients that are reactive. Tapioca is highly inflammatory, with a high glycemic index. Potato starch is the most inflammatory component of potatoes. Xanthan gum, a thickening agent, is often included as well. It is high in purines, which affect uric acid levels, which in turn can aggravate pain and inflammation. We know that when foods trigger inflammatory diseases, an uptick on the scale always follows.

(continued)

Dan's body responded fantastically well his first week on The Plan, so he and I decided to test him on rye. He passed with a half-pound weight loss and no digestive issues at all. On Day Eight, he was excited to try an English muffin, which he hadn't had in years. I told him to add a healthy amount of butter and email me the following morning.

The next day, Dan was up 1.4 pounds. It didn't make sense with his profile, so I asked him what kind of English muffin he'd had, and he told me it was high fiber. I then asked him to please look at the ingredient list and tell me if oat bran was there, and sure enough, that was the source of the extra fiber. Oats are 85 percent reactive. Suddenly, Dan's weight gain made sense.

Dan repeated the test on bread after taking a rest day, this time eating a plain white English muffin. This time, he lost .4 pounds. That is a classic illustration of how your weight is always your chemical response to food, and how the common food myths of "healthy" can sometimes be so very wrong for us.

UPON AWAKENING

- Weigh yourself and record the results in your Plan Journal.
- Drink 16 ounces of fresh water with lemon juice (after you weigh yourself).
- Take your liver support supplement and/or drink a cup of dandelion tea.

BREAKFAST

For women: 1 cup of flax granola with choice of approved fruit
For men: 1½ cups of flax granola with choice of approved fruit
Silk coconut milk or Rice Dream

LUNCH

Open-face sandwich (one slice of bread for women, 2 slices for men)
    with goat cheese, baby romaine, grated carrots, and avocado
Cream of Broccoli Soup (page 294)

White or Wheat?

I'm often asked if it's better to eat whole wheat bread rather than white, and the answer, surprisingly, is not really. Sorry to fly in the face of convention, but if you're eating healthfully in general and getting enough fiber—which you will on The Plan—you can go ahead and have that white bread if it makes you happy. Obviously, if you're traveling or just on the go and the only lettuce you can get is iceberg, go for the whole wheat bread. But if you have a fully balanced diet with plenty of grain and vegetable fiber, then the white bread is going to have a minimal impact.

SNACK

Katie's Kale Chips (page 211) or Plan Trail Mix (page 293)
(¼ cup for women, ½ cup for men)

DINNER

Protein that has been tested on a bed of spinach
Leftover sautéed vegetables

DESSERT

1 ounce of dark chocolate or Cinnamon Poached Fruit (page 185)
with optional Katie's Whipped Coconut Cream (page 296)

WATER

Be sure to drink your recommended daily water intake throughout the day, ending by dinner.

The Inside Scoop on Day Eight

Bread just needs to be better understood. The problem with most breads—which is why they make us feel unwell and gain weight—is that they often have added gluten in them...or contain high-reactive grains like corn or oats...or whopping amounts of sodium. Those protein-enriched breads? Extra gluten! In fact, American strains of wheat have a much higher gluten content than wheat in much of the rest of the world. Regular consumption can start to overload our digestive system; this is yet another reason why on The Plan we say you need to rotate your foods. Any food consumed too often can start to affect your health.

Gluten is the toughest part of bread to digest. The more you add, the more digestive issues you're likely to have. If you're eating bagels day after day because they're convenient or simply because you like them, you'll build up a gluten intolerance and assume—as many people do—that all bread is the problem. It's not. It's all about what's in it (or on it...).

Regular bread, cakes, and cookies are made from lower-gluten flour, so they are usually well tolerated in moderation, say two to three times per week. Pizza, pasta, and bagels, however, have a higher gluten content (up to 20 percent). Breads do cause water retention, but if it's just water weight it adds, that's not a big deal—you can eat friendly foods and/or work out the next day and lose that right away. What we have to pay attention to is digestion. Higher amounts of gluten consumed regularly will start to interfere with digestion, and that's when we start to see an effect on health and weight.

So many people proclaim bread to be a weight loss "no," but how did they come to that conclusion? Is it the bread that is the problem, or the 85 percent reactive turkey they're using between the slices? Is it the pizza dough, or is it the acidic tomato sauce or fake cheese? Is it the roll, or the veggie sub sandwich that packs a hefty 1,300 milligrams of sodium? It's not unlike the chicken and rice example I gave in Chapter Two. If people lose weight on chicken but then gain when they eat chicken with rice, they'll usually automatically assume that the rice is the problem and cut it out of their diet. But the rice isn't the problem—it's the *combination* of chicken and rice that triggers an inflammatory response and hence weight gain.

You always want to keep an eye on the sodium content of any bread that you're eating. I love baguettes, for instance, but a 2-ounce baguette can contain up to 350 milligrams of sodium. That doesn't mean you can't have baguettes; it just means you want to work them into your menus in a smart way. Remember, potassium negates sodium, so add some green leafy vegetables to that baguette sandwich to help your body process the sodium.

Sodium Splurges

To keep your sodium intake to the recommended 1,500 milligrams, it helps to get to know the sodium content of some of your favorite foods. You want to keep any food item you're ingesting to around 7 percent or less than your recommended daily allowance (RDA). Most bread is around 170 milligrams per piece, which would be around 10 percent, so have just one slice. A cup of Special K cereal has 220 milligrams, or around 15 percent, while healthier cereals will have less than 120 milligrams. I encourage you to read labels and familiarize yourself with the sodium content of foods you enjoy (packaged foods will always have the content listed on the label, and information is readily available online for most if not all foods). The more you know, the better choices you can make about how and when to work them in—or at least offset that delicious (high-sodium) grilled cheese sandwich by eating a salad packed with potassium-rich avocado.

If most of your foods are whole foods, you can't go too wrong. Yes, vegetables have sodium—a cup of Swiss chard can have 300 milligrams—but they naturally have other minerals that work in harmony for your body's absorption. But combine Swiss chard and celery root and you might see an uptick in weight and blood pressure! To learn more, the US Department of Agriculture publishes a list of sodium content in foods (called the USDA National Nutrient Database for Standard Reference) on its website, www.ars.usda.gov.

Day Nine: Rest Day

In the second week on The Plan, we slowly start cutting back on the flax granola, so that you have greater weight loss and a variety of nutrients, and to mitigate any potential hormonal response. Every food has health benefits and—when consumed too often—health risks, so always rotate. By this point, most people are so addicted to the flax granola's magical properties that they are loath to give it up, but rest assured: we're not losing it from your rotation! We're just adding a few other breakfast options for balance.

UPON AWAKENING

- Weigh yourself and record the results in your Plan Journal.
- Drink 16 ounces of fresh water with lemon juice (after you weigh yourself).
- Take your liver support supplement and/or drink a cup of dandelion tea.

BREAKFAST

For women: 1 cup of flax granola with approved fruit

For men: 1½ cups of flax granola with approved fruit

OR

For women: 1 cup of cereal mixed with 2 tablespoons of chia seeds and 1 ounce of sunflower seeds

For men: 2 cups of cereal mixed with 4 tablespoons of chia seeds and 1 ounce of sunflower seeds

OR

For women: 1 slice of bread with 2 tablespoons of raw almond butter and ½ piece of fruit (if you passed the bread test)

For men: 1 slice of bread with 3 to 4 tablespoons of raw almond butter and 1 whole piece of fruit (if you passed the bread test)

New Grains for Breakfast

If you passed the wheat test, you can now introduce other grains like spelt and kamut into your diet. This allows for much more variety in your choice of breakfast cereals. One of our favorite brands of cereal on The Plan is Arrowhead Mills—they're low sugar, low sodium, and delicious! If you haven't passed the wheat test, don't worry; you can always retest. But for now, stick with a rice flake cereal.

LUNCH

Sautéed kale with goat cheese, ¼ avocado, and sunflower seeds
Optional Spicy Vegetarian Soup (page 180)

SNACK

Katie's Kale Chips (page 211) or salt-free potato chips (1 ounce for women, 1½ ounces for men)
OR
The Plan Trail Mix (¼ cup for women, ½ cup for men)

DINNER

Any approved protein (make sure to rotate)
Steamed or roasted winter squash (such as butternut or zucchini) with butter, cinnamon, and black pepper (1 cup for women, 1 to 2 cups for men)
The Plan Chopped Salad (page 181)

DESSERT

1 ounce dark chocolate or Cinnamon Poached Fruit (page 185) with optional Katie's Whipped Coconut Cream (page 296)

WATER

Be sure to drink your recommended daily water intake throughout the day, ending by dinner.

The Inside Scoop on Day Nine

Rice cereals are easy to find and very well tolerated. Arrowhead Mills makes a rice flake cereal that is excellent, and also has a hot rice cereal called Rice & Shine. If you want something with a little extra sweetness to it, Barbara's Honey Rice Puffins is a fine choice.

Please be sure to avoid puffed rice cereal, as anything puffed or popped interferes with digestion (that goes for rice cakes, too, which will cause more weight gain than salt-free potato chips). And if you choose a mainstream brand cereal, please make sure to check the sodium content, as these cereals tend to be sky-high in terms of sodium levels. Ideally, a cereal's sodium content should be under 140 milligrams per cup.

Day Ten: New Protein

For the second protein test day, you can either choose a new one from the list of friendlier proteins on Day Six, or test something from the higher-reactive list below. Remember that every person's chemistry is unique, and just because something is statistically more reactive, that doesn't mean that it won't work for you. If you love it, then by all means you should test it!

UPON AWAKENING

- Weigh yourself and record the results in your Plan Journal.
- Drink 16 ounces of fresh water with lemon juice (after you weigh yourself).
- Take your liver support supplement and/or drink a cup of dandelion tea.

BREAKFAST

For women: 1 cup of cereal with approved fruit, sunflower seeds, and chia seeds

For men: 1½ cups of cereal with approved fruit, sunflower seeds, and chia seeds

OR
Blueberry Compote—Quick and Easy Version (page 291)
For women: 1 cup
For men: 1½ to 2 cups

LUNCH

The Plan Chopped Salad (page 181) with pumpkin seeds topped
with steamed or sautéed winter squash and zucchini (1 cup of
squash for women, 2 cups for men)

SNACK

For women: 1 rye cracker with 1 to 2 tablespoons of almond butter
For men: 2 to 3 rye crackers with 3 to 4 tablespoons of raw
almond butter

DINNER

Choose one new protein to test from the list below (or one from
the list on page 105):
Pork
Scallops
Sautéed kale with garlic, black pepper, and Lemon Oil (page 176)
Mixed greens with avocado and apple (make enough to have
some left over for lunch on Day Eleven)

DESSERT

1 ounce of dark chocolate or Cinnamon Poached Fruit (page 185)
with optional Katie's Whipped Coconut Cream (page 296)

WATER

Be sure to drink your recommended daily water intake throughout the day, ending by dinner.

The Inside Scoop on Day Ten

Here's everything you might want to know about the new foods being introduced on Day Ten:

Cow's cheese

Cheese…every time I say it I give a little sigh of joy. Some cheese and a glass of wine are heaven to me.

Many cheeses are high in sodium, most notably feta, so those aren't the best ones to test first. We recommend starting with fresh, unsalted mozzarella, which has proven the easiest cheese test to pass. Our delicious Healthy Chicken Parmesan (page 183) is a family favorite.

The portion size for cheese on The Plan is 1 ounce. Anytime you bump up a portion size of a tested food, it's a separate test. It's not the calories we're looking at; it could just be too much dairy, protein, sugar, or fat for your body to digest. It's entirely possible that if you do well on cheese, more than an ounce might work just fine for you. If you test cow's cheese, please have it with an approved protein.

Pork

Yes, pork is high reactive for most people, but again, if it's something you normally eat and enjoy, then you have to test it! Remember that you are now in control. If it does trigger inflammation and weight gain, then you'll have gained valuable data for your body research— and you have a handful of friendly days to return to immediately that will take the weight right back off.

My one qualifier about testing pork for the first time is that it should be fresh pork, *not* bacon or deli meat slices. Cured meats are much higher in sodium and preservatives and won't give you an accurate base line reading on your body's tolerance for pork. If you pass pork, then those things can be tests later on.

Scallops

Rich in iodine, scallops are great for thyroid health. They are the least reactive of all shellfish, so if you love shrimp, lobster, crab, and so on, scallops are a good thing to test first as your gateway shellfish. And they are remarkably easy to prepare. Just pat them dry, place them in a pan with a little olive oil and herbs, sauté on each side for three to four minutes, and add a squeeze of lemon. Yum!

Day Eleven: No Test

To reset after another protein test day, Day Eleven is a friendly-foods rest day.

UPON AWAKENING

- Weigh yourself and record the results in your Plan Journal.
- Drink 16 ounces of fresh water with lemon juice (after you weigh yourself).
- Take your liver support supplement and/or drink a cup of dandelion tea.

BREAKFAST

Flax granola with approved fruit

OR

Bread with raw almond butter and approved fruit

OR

For women: ¾ cup of cereal mixed with ¼ cup of flax granola and ½ piece of fruit

For men: 1½ cups of cereal mixed with ½ cup of flax granola and 1 whole piece of fruit

LUNCH

Leftover mixed green salad with kale and pumpkin seeds
Optional: Spicy Vegetarian Soup (page 180) or Cream of Broccoli
Soup (page 294)

SNACK

Carrots with up to 6 tablespoons of Homemade Hummus
(page 181) or raw almond butter (1 to 2 tablespoons for
women, 3 to 4 tablespoons for men)

DINNER

Any approved protein (make sure to rotate)
Vegetable Timbale (page 183; 1 cup for women, 2 cups for
men; make enough to have some left over for lunch on
Day Twelve)
Spinach salad (raw) topped with sautéed shiitake mushrooms and
Lemon Oil (page 176) (make enough to have some left over
for dinner on Day Twelve)

DESSERT

1 ounce of dark chocolate or Cinnamon Poached Fruit (page 185)
with optional Katie's Whipped Coconut Cream (page 296)

WATER

Be sure to drink your recommended daily water intake throughout the day, ending by dinner.

The Inside Scoop on Day Eleven

The expected outcome when you do a rest day is that your friendly
foods will allow your body to reset itself, cool off any inflammation, and resume losing weight. But what if that doesn't happen? It's
uncommon but it can happen. Remember, there are no days of weight
gain on The Plan that can't be explained, so let's look at the clues as
to why you might have stabilized or gained after a friendly day.

What to Look For If You've Gained Weight After a Friendly Day

- **You've had too little/too much water, or drank water three to four hours before bedtime.** Anytime your weight is up, this is always the first place to look. For every sixteen ounces less than your required amount that you drink, the body will hold on to half a pound. Overdrinking or drinking after dinner (or three to four hours before bedtime) almost always shows up on the scale as water weight.

- **You've had too much sodium.** Look through yesterday's sodium content; is there anyplace where you may have unknowingly ingested more than the recommended 1,500 milligrams? (Hint: marinades, salad dressings, packaged foods, or dining out are usually the prime suspects here.) If so, you are likely retaining water weight or exacerbated a mild reactive response to something that would otherwise have proven friendly for you.

- **You overexercised.** Exercising more than four times a week or doing extreme workouts can create a state of inflammation in the body that is counterproductive and stunts weight loss—or even causes weight gain.

- **You deviated and/or didn't have enough protein or fat.** Did you deviate from The Plan guidelines yesterday by either substituting a food or increasing a portion size on a tested food? Skimp on fat or protein intake? Or maybe swap lunch and dinner without eating all the foods listed in a specific meal? The Plan's meals are all structured to give you the right chemical balance, so deviating can unknowingly trigger a reactive response. And cutting out fat or protein will almost inevitably stall or reverse weight loss.

- **You didn't get enough sleep.** Compromising on sleep can impede weight loss and impair your body's ability to restore homeostasis. The body burns energy and calories best when you are sleeping, and lack of sleep impairs cognitive function, immunity, hormonal balance, and digestion. Several studies have cited inadequate sleep as one of the causes of the obesity problem in America. On The Plan, we have found that for every two hours of sleep the body misses, it loses .2 pounds to 1 pound less.

- **Your body has not recovered yet from prior inflammation.** If you had reactivity in the preceding days and still have constipation, your system may not yet have righted itself. Consider taking a probiotic or magnesium citrate if this is the case. Please avoid laxatives and laxative teas; they are purgative, meaning they have a very explosive effect that causes a rebound in constipation. Your body becomes dependent on them, and that's far from the goal of health on The Plan.
- **Stress.** If you're in a high-stress period, it's probably going to affect your ability to lose weight because of the cortisol flooding your system. SAM-e is an excellent remedy for stress, as is magnesium.
- **Yeast overgrowth.** Yeast overgrowth rarely causes weight gain; it's more likely to cause weight stabilization. A white coating on your tongue indicates that perhaps you've had too much natural sugar or fermented products like vinegar. Taking probiotics will get yeast overgrowth under control.
- **Hormonal factors.** Three to five days before the beginning of the menstrual cycle, many women's bodies go into a proinflammatory state—even if they're eating only friendly foods. If you notice that this pattern shows up for you, hit Pause on any testing until day one of your cycle, and the inflammatory state should subside.
- **Allergies.** Many sources cited 2012 as the worst allergy season in decades (the American College of Allergy, Asthma and Immunology and the Colorado Allergy and Asthma Center, just to name two). With record-high pollen counts, it triggered allergic reactions in at least 40-million Americans, many of whom had never had allergies before and many others who saw an increase in the number of allergens that affected them. I noticed that many of our clients had a harder time losing weight during that time, even on friendly days. It makes sense, because when your histamine levels are higher, you're in an inflamed state. If you have any allergies at all, add MSM and probiotics to allow the inflammatory process to subside and keep the allergies at bay. MSM works almost immediately, and you should be able to resume testing in a day or two.

Day Twelve: New Vegetable

Any vegetable that you haven't eaten thus far on The Plan is considered a test. We incorporate only the lowest-reactive vegetables on Days One through Eleven, and on Day Twelve, we add a new one from the list below that might fall into the higher-reactive range.

UPON AWAKENING

- Weigh yourself and record the results in your Plan Journal.
- Drink 16 ounces of fresh water with lemon juice (after you weigh yourself).
- Take your liver support supplement and/or drink a cup of dandelion tea.

BREAKFAST

For women: 1 cup of flax granola with approved fruit
For men: 1½ cups of flax granola with approved fruit
OR
Smoothie (page 174) with 1 tablespoon of chia seeds and rye cracker with raw almond butter (1 cracker for women, 3 for men)
OR
For women: 1 cup of cereal with ½ piece of fruit and 1 ounce sunflower seeds and 2 tablespoons chia seeds
For men: 1½ cups of cereal with whole fruit and 1 ounce sunflower seeds and 4 tablespoons chia seeds

The Mighty Chia Seed

Chia seeds are a great source of omega-3s and calcium and pack 10 to 15 grams of protein into just 4 to 6 tablespoons. Like flaxseeds, when they get wet they form mucilage, which does an amazing job of sweeping your intestines and keeping your digestive system healthy. Plus, they add a nice little crunch. Feel free to add chia seeds to your soups, salads, smoothies, or other dishes whenever you like.

LUNCH

Leftover Vegetable Timbale (1 cup for women, 2 cups for men)
    and mixed greens with pumpkin seeds
Optional: soup of choice

SNACK

Katie's Kale Chips (page 211) or rye crackers with Homemade
    Hummus (page 181)

DINNER

Any approved protein (make sure to rotate)
Choose one new vegetable from the list below to test, to be
    mixed in with an already approved vegetable:
Snow peas
Bok choy
Brussels sprouts
Savoy cabbage
Tomatoes
Red pepper
Potato
Radicchio
Endive

*Note: When testing a new vegetable, we always include an approved
vegetable in that meal as well, to cut down on the chance of reactivity.*
Leftover spinach salad

DESSERT

1 ounce of dark chocolate or Cinnamon Poached Fruit (page 185)
    with optional Katie's Whipped Coconut Cream (page 296)

WATER

Be sure to drink your recommended daily water intake through-
    out the day, ending by dinner.

The Inside Scoop on Day Twelve

Here's what you might want to know about the vegetable choices for Day Twelve:

Snow peas

Snow peas are a great gateway test for green beans, snap peas, and peanut butter, as they are the least reactive vegetable in that family. For the first test, the portion size is the smallest amount possible, say five to six peapods.

Bok choy, Brussels sprouts, Savoy cabbage

These are easier tests than other crucifers like cauliflower. Serving sizes for bok choy and Savoy cabbage are ½ cup; for Brussels sprouts, limit the first test to four or five (cut them in half before cooking and it will feel like much more).

Tomatoes

I recommend beginning with one plum tomato. Plum tomatoes work beautifully in the Healthy Chicken Parmesan recipe (page 183), which many people love. Please save grape or cherry tomatoes for a future test, as they are higher in acidity.

Red bell pepper

Please be sure to test on red peppers first rather than green, orange, or yellow. Green peppers are simply unripe red ones, and they cause more digestive issues.

Potato

You can choose half a regular potato or one smaller potato (purple, fingerling, etc). Baked or roasted is fine, and as with any vegetable, potatoes test best when eaten along with other vegetables. The problem with potatoes comes in when people eat huge quantities or make them their main course. One of the most popular dishes among Plan people is Roasted Italian Winter Vegetables (page 184) with potatoes.

> ### Butter on Vegetables? Yes!
>
> Butter is an excellent source of vitamin D, and the all-important fat, which keeps you satiated, ensures healthy brain function, and fortifies the phospholipid barrier in your cell walls. Plus, butter tastes *delicious* melted on cooked vegetables!

Day Thirteen: No Test

Day Thirteen is another rest day. I encourage you to follow each rest day's menu as it is laid out. The more rest days you do well on, the more your body is encouraged to heal.

UPON AWAKENING

- Weigh yourself and record the results in your Plan Journal.
- Drink 16 ounces of fresh water with lemon juice (after you weigh yourself).
- Take your liver support supplement and/or drink a cup of dandelion tea.

BREAKFAST

For women: 1 cup of flax granola with approved fruit
For men: 1½ cups of flax granola with approved fruit
OR
Smoothie (page 174) with chia seeds and rye cracker with raw almond butter (1 cracker with 1 to 2 tablespoons of raw almond butter for women, 2 crackers with 3 to 4 tablespoons of raw almond butter for men)

LUNCH

(Reheated) leftover vegetables on a bed of baby romaine with goat cheese and sunflower seeds

Choice of soup

OR

Approved salad (mixed greens, spinach salad, kale salad, etc.)
   with a minimum of 15 grams of vegetarian protein of your
   choice (with the exception of rice) and soup of choice

Vegetarian Sources of Protein

In Part Three, you'll learn how to construct your own chemically balanced test and rest days. In anticipation of that, now is a good time
to start becoming familiar with the protein content of easily digested
protein sources:

- Broccoli: 5 grams per cup
- Sunflower seeds: 5 grams per ounce
- Pumpkin seeds: 9 grams per ounce
- Almonds: 8 grams per ounce
- Cheese: 8 grams per ounce
- Chickpeas: 5 grams per ½ cup
- Chia seeds: 5 grams per 2 tablespoons
- Rice: 5 grams per cup
- Hemp seeds: 8 grams per 2 tablespoons.

SNACK

Salt-free potato chips (1 ounce for women, 1½ ounces for men)

OR

The Plan Trail Mix (¼ cup for women, ½ cup for men)

DINNER

Approved protein (make sure to rotate) on a bed of mixed greens

Roasted Italian Winter Vegetables (page 184; 1 to 2 cups for
   women, 2 to 3 cups for men. You can add any new vegetable
   you tested and passed on Day Twelve; make enough to have
   leftovers for lunch on Day Fourteen)

DESSERT

1 ounce of dark chocolate or Cinnamon Poached Fruit (page 185) with optional Katie's Whipped Coconut Cream (page 296)

WATER

Be sure to drink your recommended daily water intake throughout the day, ending by dinner.

Day Fourteen: Test New Breakfast Addition (or Milk)

Day Fourteen is a favorite for many people because it's a chance to try out some breakfast options that they love. It's all about choosing something you ordinarily enjoy. Oatmeal, yogurt, French toast, a bagel with butter...it's up to you. You already know a lot about your body's responses to different foods, and this is a great chance to start putting that into practice. If you tested reactive to bread, French toast probably isn't the best choice. But if you passed bread, then by all means, go for it. If you tested eggs and gained .8 pound, then perhaps pass on the omelet with goat cheese and herbs and try a new cereal instead.

Alternatively, you can use today to test whole or lactose-free milk. If you love lattes, today's the day to test one. Or if you prefer regular milk on your cereal rather than rice or coconut milk, give it a try.

Please just be sure to stick to *one* test today to make sure we get accurate results. If you're testing whole milk on cereal, test it with an already approved cereal. If you're testing a bagel but haven't tested cow's cheese yet, skip the cream cheese and go with butter instead. If you love sprouted-grain bread and want to test it, toast up a piece with raw almond butter if almonds have proven friendly for you. Testing your favorite diner for breakfast? Go with an already-known friendly food (for more guidance on testing restaurants, please see Day Eighteen). You get the picture.

UPON AWAKENING

- Weigh yourself and record the results in your Plan Journal.
- Drink 16 ounces of fresh water with lemon juice (after you weigh yourself).
- Take your liver support supplement and/or drink a cup of dandelion tea.

BREAKFAST

Test new breakfast item
OR
Whole or lactose-free milk

The Egg-and-Bread Combo

In Part Three, you'll learn the food combinations that are specific tests (for instance, chicken and rice). One that might apply to today's test, however, is a favorite breakfast combo: eggs and bread. Sadly, this is typically a high-reactive combo, but as you've heard me say enough times by now: if you love it, you should test it. Eggs Benedict fans, I have my fingers crossed for you!

LUNCH

Roasted Italian Winter Vegetables (page 184; 1 cup for women, 2 to 3 cups for men) on a bed of spinach with goat cheese
Rye cracker with Homemade Hummus (page 181; 1 cracker for women, 2 crackers for men)

SNACK

For women: ½ piece of approved fruit and a small handful of raw almonds
For men: 1 whole piece of fruit and a small handful of raw almonds

DINNER

Approved protein (make sure to rotate)

Leftover Winter Vegetables from dinner on Day Thirteen

Sautéed zucchini and broccoli with basil, Lemon Oil (page 176),
and 1 tablespoon grated Manchego (make enough to have
some left over for lunch on Day Fifteen)

DESSERT

1 ounce of dark chocolate or Cinnamon Poached Fruit (page 185)
with optional Katie's Whipped Coconut Cream (page 296)

WATER

Be sure to drink your recommended daily water intake throughout the day, ending by dinner.

Why Does It Seem Like I'm Reactive to Everything?

For some people, everything seems to test reactive. This can be
incredibly frustrating, but there's always a reason behind it. One of
the biggest factors that can hinder success on The Plan is leaky gut
syndrome, otherwise known as increased intestinal permeability.
Leaky gut can be attributed to years of eating foods that are inflammatory and other factors like NSAIDs such as Advil and Motrin, candida, and environmental toxins.

Here's what happens: your intestines have a mucosal barrier that
keeps bacteria, antigens, and undigested food from leaking through.
Normally this barrier is pretty tight, but when you eat a reactive food
or are ingesting irritating substances, it can start to loosen the junctures, known as desmosomes. If this isn't addressed by omitting the
reactive agents, the junctures get more and more permeable, and
undigested foods can now go directly into your bloodstream. Your
body recognizes them as invaders and starts to prepare a defense,

using antibodies and lymphocytes to deal with the particles that just shouldn't be there; this is an inflammatory response. The more often this happens, the weaker your digestion becomes, until eventually even the friendliest foods can trigger gas, bloating, and constipation. There are, of course, other problems that can develop when this is left untreated, like stress on the liver and immune system, so the sooner we take care of this the better!

Finding and eliminating your reactive foods and cutting out excess alcohol and medications is key (though please always check with your doctor before ceasing any medication). For nutritional support, you can take probiotics and MSM and consult with a medical and/or holistic practitioner.

Day Fifteen: No Test

This is another rest day to add to your friendly-day repertoire.

UPON AWAKENING

- Weigh yourself and record the results in your Plan Journal.
- Drink 16 ounces of fresh water with lemon juice (after you weigh yourself).
- Take your liver support supplement and/or drink a cup of dandelion tea.

BREAKFAST

Smoothie (page 174) with chia seeds, rye cracker, and nut butter
OR
Flax granola and approved fruit

LUNCH

Sandwich with leftover zucchini, cheese, and sunflower
    seeds
Mixed greens or soup of choice

OR

Approved salad with a minimum of 15 grams of vegetarian protein
and soup of choice (20 grams of vegetarian protein for men)

SNACK

Carrots with 1 to 2 tablespoons of raw almond butter

DINNER

Chicken with Indian Spice Rub (page 174)

Sautéed Kale with Vegetables (page 178; make enough to have
some left over for lunch on Day Sixteen)

Steamed broccoli with lemon and Lemon Oil (page 176) (make
enough to have some left over for dinner on Day Sixteen)

DESSERT

1 ounce of dark chocolate or Cinnamon Poached Fruit (page 185)
with optional Katie's Whipped Coconut Cream (page 296)

WATER

Be sure to drink your recommended daily water intake throughout the day, ending by dinner.

If Weight Loss Stalls

When your body starts to consistently lose weight in .2-pound incre-
ments instead of .5, there is a good chance that you are reaching a
set point. Certainly if your body stays at the exact same number with
no deviation at all for four straight days, that is a sign that you have
reached a point where your body is saying, "No more weight loss,
please."

Most people have a pretty good idea of what their set point is.
What has your optimal weight been in your lifetime? When did you
feel your best? If you were at that weight while living a healthy lifestyle (meaning no extreme dieting, fasting, stress, illness, etc.), then

that's your set point. If you were rail-thin on a yeast-free, 1,000-calorie-a-day diet, that's not a realistic weight goal—or a way to live and enjoy life. Some people worry about becoming too skinny on The Plan, but it just doesn't happen. It's too healthy a diet in terms of balance and calories, and your body will naturally regulate itself.

If you have a lot of weight to lose and you lose very rapidly at first, you may hit a plateau. We've seen this with our clients who have 100 pounds or more to lose. The first 50 pounds come off easily, but after that, they hit a little roadblock. The first instinct when the scale doesn't budge is usually "Oh no! Eat less!" because we've been programmed that way. But that's actually the worst thing you can do. Just keep eating normally according to The Plan's guidelines and your body will realize it is not in starvation mode and once again resume weight loss.

Day Sixteen: Two Proteins in One Day

Having animal protein twice in one day is a test, which we do on Day Sixteen. We do a half portion at lunch the first time, to minimize the chance of reactivity. By way of reminder, a full portion of chicken, beef, pork, etc., is 4 to 6 ounces for women and 6 to 8 ounces for men.

UPON AWAKENING

- Weigh yourself and record the results in your Plan Journal.
- Drink 16 ounces of fresh water with lemon juice (after you weigh yourself).
- Take your liver support supplement and/or drink a cup of dandelion tea.

BREAKFAST

Flax granola with approved fruit
OR
New approved breakfast

LUNCH

Leftover Sautéed Kale with Vegetables with 2 ounces of chicken
with Indian Spice Rub (page 174)
Rye cracker with cheese (1 cracker for women, 3 crackers for
men)

SNACK

For women: ½ piece of fruit with almonds
For men: 1 whole piece of fruit with almonds

DINNER

Approved protein (make sure to rotate) on a bed of mixed greens
Sautéed or steamed approved vegetable

DESSERT

1 ounce of dark chocolate or Cinnamon Poached Fruit (page 185)
with optional Katie's Whipped Coconut Cream (page 296)

WATER

Be sure to drink your recommended daily water intake throughout the day, ending by dinner.

The Inside Scoop on Day Sixteen

On the day(s) when you incorporate animal protein for lunch, pay
attention to your energy levels in the afternoon. Do you feel an
energy dip a few hours after lunch? This is something we see very
often. If so, it indicates that your body does better with vegetarian
protein sources midday.

As ever, that doesn't mean you *can't* have animal protein at lunch.
It simply means that you have the information about that in hand and
can make informed choices about if, when, and how to work it in. A
favorite lunch for my client Mark is a big salad with grilled chicken.

But like so many people, when Mark tested chicken at lunch during the work day, he had an energy lull at 3 p.m. So he switched things up a bit and now saves his beloved grilled chicken salads for the weekends, when 3 p.m. is prime rest and relaxation time for him. All it takes is having the data in hand and a little creative thinking, and most of your favorite foods can continue to be a joyful part of your life.

Day Seventeen: No Test

UPON AWAKENING

- Weigh yourself and record the results in your Plan Journal.
- Drink 16 ounces of fresh water with lemon juice (after you weigh yourself).
- Take your liver support supplement and/or drink a cup of dandelion tea.

BREAKFAST

Flax granola with approved fruit

LUNCH

Spicy Chickpea Spinach Salad (page 180; make enough to have some left over for lunch on Day Eighteen)

Butternut Squash Soup (page 182; make enough to have some left over for lunch on Day Eighteen)

SNACK

Rye cracker with raw almond butter (1 cracker for women, 3 crackers for men)

DINNER

Approved protein (make sure to rotate) on a bed of mixed greens

Vegetable Timbale (page 183; 1 cup for women, 2 cups for
men; make enough to have some left over for dinner on
Day Nineteen)

DESSERT

1 ounce of dark chocolate or Cinnamon Poached Fruit (page 185)
with optional Katie's Whipped Coconut Cream (page 296)

WATER

Be sure to drink your recommended daily water intake throughout the day, ending by dinner.

Day Eighteen: Test a New Restaurant

A key part of The Plan is learning how to dine at your favorite places
and be healthy and easily attain or maintain your goal weight. Today
you'll learn the easy protocol for testing restaurants.

UPON AWAKENING

- Weigh yourself and record the results in your Plan Journal.
- Drink 16 ounces of fresh water with lemon juice (after you
  weigh yourself).
- Take your liver support supplement and/or drink a cup of dandelion tea.

BREAKFAST

Flax granola with approved fruit
OR
Flax granola with approved cereal and approved fruit
OR
Smoothie with chia seeds and rye cracker with nut butter
(1 cracker for women, 3 crackers for men)
OR
New approved breakfast

LUNCH

Salad with 15 grams of protein (20 grams for men)

Choice of approved soup

SNACK

For women: 1 ounce of salt-free potato chips and ⅛ cup of
Homemade Guacamole (page 204)

For men: 1½ ounces of salt-free potato chips and ¼ cup of
Homemade Guacamole (page 204)

DINNER

Test a restaurant

OR

If you are not dining out on Day Eighteen, you can test a new
vegetable. The dinner menu would be:

Any approved protein (make sure to rotate)

Any salad

And test a new cooked vegetable

DESSERT

Crème brûlée, chocolate desserts, biscotti, and, of course, fruit
with whipped cream are all relatively safe desserts. To get the
best read on your body's response to the restaurant you've
chosen, you can share a dessert with a dining companion.

The Real Scoop on Ice Cream

The dessert that can cause the most damage after a meal is ice cream.
One problem is dairy overload. In addition, anything cold inhibits
digestion, and whenever we do that we are asking for trouble. If you
love ice cream, I recommend saving it for an afternoon snack on a
nice hot day.

(continued)

Whole ingredients will always burn cleanest for your body, so go for the gelato, not the Skinny Cow. Gelato is quite simply "clean ice cream," and by that I mean it's made with simple ingredients your grandmother would use: milk, cream, eggs, sugar, and, of course, whatever individual flavors are used, like chocolate, vanilla, strawberries, etc. Luckily for consumers, the tide is turning toward healthier options. Häagen-Dazs now has a product called Five, and that's it—just five ingredients! Remember, the fewer chemicals and preservatives, the better your body can digest.

WATER

Be sure to drink your recommended daily water intake throughout the day.

Note: This is especially important on restaurant testing days to mitigate sodium intake.

The Inside Scoop on Day Eighteen

Here is everything you might want to know about testing a new restaurant, to make dining out a successful and happy experience:

Stick with Your Tested Friendly Foods

The restaurant itself is the test, so you don't want to throw in another variable to confuse the data. It's best to stay with foods you have already tested at home to minimize weight gain and negative health reactions. If you tested well on steak, by all means go ahead and order that filet mignon. If scallops, pork chops, or lamb worked well for you, choose those. The same goes for potatoes, green beans, tomatoes, or anything else, staying with your normal portion sizes for everything. One caveat: while chicken is majorly Plan friendly when prepared at home, at restaurants I don't advise it because chicken masks the taste of sodium so well.

If you stabilize or gain after dining out, remember: that's okay.

You're in control! If you stuck with your friendly foods, then the weight gain is just water weight as a result of the excess sodium and will be relatively easy to flush out the following day with a friendly-foods day.

If none of your friendly foods are on the menu, don't panic. Just order what makes the most sense and try a half portion of the new food rather than the full order. Surround the restaurant meal with foods that are friendly for you and make sure you're properly hydrated. If you do gain, you can relax, knowing that tomorrow you'll do a rest day with your friendly foods and bounce right back. That's the beauty of The Plan long-term.

Dine by the Golden Sodium Rule

I absolutely love dining out. What I don't love is waking up the next day with a puffy face from all the sodium. I'll never understand why restaurants insist on oversalting everything! And it's not just fast-food establishments we're talking about, where a burger can have 6,000 milligrams of sodium. Some of the finest restaurants in the country have a heavy hand when it comes to the salt.

But that doesn't mean you have to accept it. While there isn't much we can do about the salt added to fast food, if you're dining in a regular restaurant—regardless of whether it's casual or high end—you can always ask them to prepare your food without added salt. The Plan's Golden Sodium Rule is simple: *If it tastes salty, send it back!*

Here's a tip that many of my clients use: if you're going someplace where you know you'll be ordering meat, which is usually pre-seasoned with lots of salt, call ahead of time and ask if they can set aside a piece without marinade for you. Better restaurants will accommodate you, as long as you ask before you go (they won't do it midservice, since they'll be in the thick of the cooking and serving rush). And if they won't grant your request when you call in advance, then at least you'll know the level to which that restaurant is Plan-friendly.

Wine, by the way, goes a long way toward mitigating the effects of the added salt in restaurant foods. Because it is a diuretic, it helps flush out sodium, and it also aids digestion. I also like to have a little predinner snack of salt-free potato chips and guacamole, both high in potassium, which counteracts sodium.

Enjoy yourself

Ellen, sixty-one, was doing beautifully on The Plan. She came to me with acid reflux and forty pounds to lose. By Day Eighteen, her acid reflux was essentially gone and she'd dropped nine pounds. Ellen's husband, Jeff, was completely supportive of her efforts, and knowing that Day Eighteen was her restaurant testing day, he planned a special dinner at their favorite restaurant.

Ellen and Jeff had a wonderful time. They drank wine, talked, laughed, and enjoyed a delicious meal. It wasn't until early the next morning that Ellen started worrying about the portion size of her steak (it was bigger than she normally had), the sodium in the marinade, the whole baked potato she'd had, the slice of pie she and Jeff had shared for dessert. Certain that she'd gained weight, Ellen stepped on the scale the next morning and saw that she hadn't gained a single ounce.

How did that happen? Simple. On The Plan we call it the joy factor. We are social creatures by nature. When we allow ourselves to revel in the joy of dining—lingering over meals, savoring, laughing, and concentrating on the friendship and banter as much as the food—our bodies respond in kind. I can't tell you how many clients I've had who told me they went to a cocktail party and laughed their heads off and indulged in all kinds of treats, and yet didn't gain a pound. Joy is a major ingredient in long-term health and weight loss success on The Plan—and in life.

So please, enjoy yourself. Test a restaurant you love with people who make you smile, and *relax*. I insist!

Best Restaurant Choices

The restaurants where you can most easily find Plan-friendly foods are New American and Italian restaurants. Additionally, any restaurant that calls itself "new" or "modern" will generally make lighter and healthier interpretations of ethnic cuisines. There you can usually find Plan staples of proteins with vegetables and wonderful spices and a salad. You can always play it safe and order a plain grilled protein if you are worried about the sauces and sodium.

If sushi is a favorite of yours, as it is for many people, the best way to test a restaurant is to have sashimi with brown rice. (Please note much of the fish in sushi restaurants is farm-raised). Brown rice usually works much better than the regular sushi rice, which is very starchy and causes water retention. Add just a dash of soy sauce mixed with water and wasabi for flavor, if you normally enjoy those. The pickled ginger is high in sodium and often has MSG, so just limit consumption.

The food at Chinese restaurants tends to be very high in sodium. I have many clients who cook traditional Chinese food at home and lose weight consistently. They order from a restaurant and *bam*, sodium weight gain. Of all the Asian cuisines, Thai usually has the least MSG and sodium.

Mexican food is superfun, but unfortunately not a sure-fire weight loss meal in much of the United States. The staples of Mexican food, like corn, black beans, and salsa, are problematic for many, and much of the food is high in sodium. Certainly a couple of safer bets would be ceviche and guacamole. Try to find restaurants that specialize in regional cuisine; it's closer to the foods as they are prepared in Mexico, and most people I've worked with do lose weight when they eat at restaurants like those.

Annika, 43

I feel like I have finally arrived home after a journey of a thousand miles. For years I have been struggling to understand why I seem to gain weight easily and why it has been so very difficult to lose. I finally have the answers to my questions now! I can relax and know that what I am eating is the best food for me. No more *"What should I order…I wonder if this food will make me gain weight?"* Through my involvement in The Plan, I know which foods help me to lose weight and which foods I can look forward to having as a treat. Even wine and chocolate are on the list! Furthermore, it's so easy to stay on The Plan because there are absolutely no cravings when your system is in balance.

It's great to know that not only have I lost weight but I am so much healthier than I was previously. My bad cholesterol levels have been reduced tremendously, and my doctor said she was so impressed with my results. I remember when I started The Plan at the end of December, thinking it would be a great way to ring in the new year. Now, three months later and fifteen pounds lighter, I see I was absolutely right!

Day Nineteen: Test New Vegetable

Just a reminder: the best way to test a new vegetable is to mix it in with other vegetables that are already tested and friendly for you, to cut down on the potential for reactivity. If your weight is up from yesterday's test, you may switch days Nineteen and Twenty.

UPON AWAKENING

- Weigh yourself and record the results in your Plan Journal.
- Drink 16 ounces of fresh water with lemon juice (after you weigh yourself).
- Take your liver support supplement and/or drink a cup of dandelion tea.

BREAKFAST

Flax granola with approved fruit

OR

For women: 1 cup of cereal with sunflower and chia seeds and
½ piece of fruit

For men: 1½ cups of cereal with sunflower seeds and chia seeds
and 1 whole piece of fruit

LUNCH

Leftover Vegetable Timbale (1 cup for women, 2 cups for men) on
a bed of spinach with pumpkin seeds

Spicy Vegetarian Soup (page 180)

SNACK

Rye crackers (1 for women, 2 for men) 1 to 2 tablespoons of raw
almond butter

OR

The Plan Trail Mix (page 293; ¼ cup for women, ½ cup for men)

DINNER

Any approved protein (make sure ti rotate)

Add a new vegetable to vegetable sauté

Arugula with diced pear

DESSERT

1 ounce of dark chocolate or Cinnamon Poached Fruit (page 185)
with optional Katie's Whipped Coconut Cream (page 296)

WATER

Be sure to drink your recommended daily water intake throughout the day, ending by dinner.

Day Twenty: No Test

On Day Twenty, you can repeat any of your favorite days thus far that yielded the most weight loss and best health responses.

Completing Your Twenty Days

This is just the beginning, my friends. I would imagine that by now you are well on your way to your weight loss goal, and hopefully your health concerns are markedly improved—if not gone altogether.

In Part Three, we're going to move on to Phase Three of The Plan, which is learning to test on your own. Trust me: you're ready!

Eleanor, 62

I'm one of those people who has dieted my entire life. You name a diet and I've tried it. I would lose weight initially, but eventually it would all return, plus more. I needed to lose weight for my health. In addition to having a few inflammation-based conditions (lupus, asthma, eczema, arthritis, macular degeneration), my cholesterol was high and my blood pressure was slowly creeping up to unsafe levels. To my regimen of vitamins and prescription drugs the doctor added cholesterol and high blood pressure medicine.

Frustrated and unhappy with myself, I decided I had to do something else. My son told me about The Plan. Working with Lyn-Genet for a month, I learned to "listen" to my body and see how it reacts to food. With her guidance, I learned what foods were good for me to eat and how to test foods at a future date.

A sweet tooth was something I'd always had, but with The Plan, I don't crave sugar like I used to. Fruit is the sweetness I need, instead of cake and candy. Eating seeds, nuts, and dried fruit has controlled my appetite. Learning combinations of foods that cause weight gain was also important to my weight loss. Drinking water was never something I enjoyed. Learning how to calculate the amount of water I should drink and how it changes as you gain or lose weight was very enlightening.

After following The Plan for three months, I went to a scheduled checkup with my doctor. My cholesterol had been at 173 with medicine; after three months on The Plan, it went down to 147. My doctor said he was shocked. He had never seen anyone's cholesterol numbers go down so much in such a short time. I no longer need the medicine. He even asked me for the name of my nutritionist so that he could recommend her to other patients!

I continue to use The Plan and lose weight. There are fewer aches and pains and no bloating. I feel terrific! The Plan makes me feel confident that the knowledge I have gained will help me keep the weight off and help me be a healthier person.

Part Three

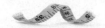

THE PLAN FOR LIFE

CHAPTER SIX

Phase Three—Testing on Your Own

The Plan doesn't end after your twenty days. Far from it! Everything you've learned thus far about how your body processes different foods lays the foundation for a lifetime of eating healthfully—the *real*, sustainable version of healthy and slim. And now, in Phase Three, I'm going to teach you all the formulas and secrets you need to know to build your own balanced menu plans for test days and rest days going forward, so you can have a system that works for life.

Testing New Foods

The most direct path to losing weight is to follow the easy basics of constructing balanced daily menus and to find forty to fifty foods that are friendly for your body. Learn and do both of those things and you'll get to your goal weight. Even better, you'll know exactly how to stay there.

I've said this before, but it's worth repeating: it can be tempting to just park yourself in the friendly-foods zone after your initial twenty days, because you know what works and how to lose weight easily. But I really encourage you not to stop testing; otherwise, your body will adapt and your weight loss efforts will stall. In addition, you may create food sensitivities if you don't keep rotating and adding in new foods.

Take Holly, forty-four, for example. Holly went through her twenty-day Plan, established her friendly foods, and lost twelve pounds. After she went out on her own, she didn't want to test and risk weight gain. But the whole idea is that you keep testing, you keep adding new things. She emailed me to check in, and when I heard that her weight loss had been stalling on friendly days, I knew right away what was going on. I tough-loved Holly into resuming her testing, and she averaged a weight loss of .8 pound daily for two weeks straight before settling back into a steady .5-pound loss daily.

When you test a new food, yes, you always run the risk of gaining, but you need to go through this process so you can establish a large list of friendly foods that you can enjoy and rotate without thinking about whether or not you'll gain. Growing pains is what I call it. You'll need to find several proteins that work for you and keep cycling them in and out throughout the week for proper weight loss. Staying with the same foods day in and day out will not only create mind-numbing boredom, it will lead to slower weight loss and inadequate nutrition. I cannot stress this enough: *continuing to test in Phase Three of The Plan is essential for long-term success.* So go ahead and experiment and expand your food horizons.

Guidelines for Testing New Foods

- For greater weight loss, it's best to test a new food every four to five days. That way, if the food turns out to be reactive, you have enough friendly days in between to still have adequate weight loss until you get to your goal weight.

- When designing a test day, use only ingredients (including spices and condiments) that you've used before and add only *one* new ingredient or food to the day. Surround every new test food with friendly foods so you'll immediately identify reactivity if it happens. (I'll go into more specifics about daily menus in a moment. I'll give you the basic formula below, and you'll just plug in the variables.)

- Proper hydration is a must. Anytime you had a drop in weight these past twenty days, you had friendly foods and proper hydration (not too little and not too much). You won't have one without the other in that formula.

- When you're testing something new, you always want to test in the smallest reasonable amount to see what your body can tolerate. With something that's generally low reactive, you can be a little more liberal (you can always refer to the chart titled "Potential Reactivity of Foods" on page 81 for a refresher), but if you're testing mustard, say, or corn, try a small amount the first time. Might as well minimize the effects if it does in fact prove reactive for you!

- Though it may be tempting to cut calories so you can "pass" a new food test, I encourage you not to. Sure, if you limit your food intake and calories enough on a testing day, you can pass the test on practically anything. But that's not realistic testing; when you have that food on a normal day with normal caloric intake, your response will likely vary. So keep it real and test a new food sensibly.

- Test what's important to you and what you enjoy. You want to test frozen yogurt? Test frozen yogurt. Vodka? Go for it. There's no "wrong" thing to test. If that's what you love, then that's what you're going to want, so you might as well test it! I'm not here to judge you on what you want to incorporate into your life. If these are things you eat or drink on a regular basis, they're what you need to test.

- Remember that any portion size of a friendly food that is increased by more than, say, 15 to 20 percent is a test. So if you tested well on one slice of bread, two slices would be another test. Half an avocado rather than a quarter is a test, as is more than half a cup of low-sodium chickpeas or a bigger cut of steak or other protein than what you've been having on The Plan. Simply test the bigger portion size on its own, the same as you would a new food.

- Certain food combinations are tests as well. The potentially problematic combos to watch out for and be sure to test before assuming they're okay (even if both components are already friendly for your body on their own) are:

Rice and beans in the same meal
Rice and animal protein in the same meal
Beans and meat in the same meal
Eggs and another animal protein in the same day

Planning Your Own Menus

Some clients tell me they feel apprehensive as they approach their twenty-day mark. They worry about whether they've learned enough to construct their own menus, how they'll know if they're getting it right, whether they'll be able to read their body's signals. I tell them the same thing I'm telling you: *relax and trust yourself*! You know more than you think you do.

You certainly know by this point how to read your body's signals, and if you get confused, you can go back again and again to read through the methodology laid out in Part Two. And I promise, it's easy to create balanced daily menus for both testing and resting days once you know the basics. If you follow the basic guidelines laid out below, you pretty much can't go wrong.

Guidelines for Daily Menu Plans

- **Protein:** You want to aim for at least 10 grams of protein at breakfast, 15 to 40 at lunch, 40 to 70 at dinner. (Please see sidebars for the protein content of common protein sources.) Remember how much weight you were losing that first week on The Plan? You were consuming 80 to 100 grams of protein, so don't think that eating just greens with tomato and cucumber is going to do the trick! I know it's counterintuitive, but I can't tell you how many people stall weight loss by just having mixed greens with no protein for lunch.

- It's also essential to rotate your friendly proteins. Here are some rough guidelines to follow. You may be able to tolerate more or less, and soon you'll come up with your own template, the one that will work best for your body.

> **Steak:** best to have only once every seven days
> **Lamb:** two to three times weekly
> **Beans:** once per day
> **Fish:** twice weekly
> **Eggs:** once every other day (daily is a separate test)
> **Nuts and seeds:** 1 to 2 servings of nuts and 1 to 2 servings
>   of seeds per day
> **Cheese:** 1 to 2 ounces per day

- **Vegetables:** Include as many as you can fit into a day from the list of vegetables we have used thus far, as well as any that you have tested well on. Steaming and sautéing are ideal; roasting concentrates natural sugars. If yeast is an issue, limit roasted vegetables and squash to 1 cup several times a week.
- **Fresh fruit:** All fruits other than the ones you've incorporated thus far on The Plan are a test. A classic diet mistake is to eat tons of fruit, thinking it's healthy, but too much fruit overloads your body with natural sugar. Limit fresh fruit to no more than one and a half or two servings per day.
- **Dense carbs (rice, pasta, bread):** One serving per day is best for weight loss for most people. Remember that a dense carb and a protein eaten in the same meal are a separate test (for instance, beans and rice or chicken with pasta; fish and rice tends to be the easiest mix for most people).
- **Condiments and sauces:** Condiments like ketchup and mustard, salad dressings, and sauces that you have not already tested,

like barbecue sauce, tomato sauce, etc., are all tests. Use them on a food you've tested and passed and/or on a Plan-approved low-reactive food, and make sure that's your one new addition that day to determine whether it is friendly for you.

- **Herbs and Spices:** Spices are your best friend when it comes to cooking! Try to include cumin, cinnamon, cayenne, turmeric, and ginger (all anti-inflammatory spices) in your food as often as you can for flavoring, and test others that you like. Try growing herbs on your windowsill. They are a wonderful, bright addition to meals. I always encourage parents to have their children help take care of the herb plants. Smelling them will develop the kids' palates early for fresh vegetables!
- **Sweets and treats:** Remember, everything is a test. If you have a favorite dessert, candy, or other treat that you want to incorporate into your life, by all means test it!

The bottom line is this: if you're not sure whether something is a test, just program it in on a friendly day and try it out. But please don't drive yourself crazy—this isn't about being perfect! You have the data and tools you need at your disposal now, and you'll very soon become adept at reading and tweaking the variables as necessary.

Protein Contents

- Sunflower seeds: 5 grams per ounce
- Pumpkin seeds: 9 grams per ounce
- Almonds: 8 grams per ounce
- Cheese: 8 grams per ounce
- Chickpeas: 5 grams per ½ cup
- Chia seeds: 5 grams per 2 tablespoons
- Rice: 5 grams per cup
- Animal protein: approximately 7 grams per ounce (reminder: keep the balance of your animal proteins programmed in at dinner rather than lunch until you test how your body responds otherwise)

Rayna, 49

I love The Plan and how I feel—it's what I've been looking for, for a long time! I have struggled with my weight and health issues for several years. I would lose weight on programs and then gain all of it back or more. I had high cholesterol and, according to blood tests, was prediabetic.

It makes sense that everyone's body reacts to different foods and that different foods cause different people to gain weight. On The Plan, I have been surprised to learn what my body reacts to. I'd been eating several of those foods for years; when I stopped eating them, the weight came off quickly and consistently. I have been thrilled that my cholesterol has gone down 120 points in less than two months, and I'm no longer prediabetic.

I love that The Plan is manageable and can be done for the rest of my life. I never feel deprived or hungry. I know if I have a "bad" day the weight will come off if I just get back on The Plan and eat my friendly foods. It is definitely worth the effort, time, and commitment to make my life the life I always wanted it to be.

CHAPTER SEVEN

The Plan Lifestyle

The Plan, as you already well know, isn't a diet. During Phase One and Phase Two, when you are actively testing new foods to get to a solid forty to fifty that work for you, it is a standardized protocol. After that, it becomes a very natural and easy way of life.

> Rebecca, 43
>
> The Plan helps keep everything in balance. I've certainly gone off The Plan when on vacation or some days during the weekend. I've learned two things from when that happens: one is that since I'm eating so cleanly, when I do diverge, it has a minimal or no effect because my body is in an anti-inflammatory state. The other is that if I do gain some weight, I have the tools to take it right off.

Daily Life on The Plan

A lot of clients ask about templates for working The Plan into their life going forward, and really, your life should be what dictates your Plan—not the other way around. Life isn't rigid, and neither should your eating be.

If you want to follow The Plan during the week and take the weekends off to indulge, you can do that. That's what my client Richard, forty-four, does. He has two young sons, and his weekends are action packed, with baseball games, soccer tournaments, pizza pit stops in between to celebrate wins, and family barbecues. So one weekend day is set aside as a free-for-all, and one day he makes sure to make a family favorite from The Plan recipes, like the Lamb Burgers (page 184) or the Healthy Chicken Parmesan (page 183). The dishes from The Plan are family friendly and everyone enjoys the food, so it doesn't feel like a diet.

Everyone finds their own balance on The Plan. The weight loss and health benefits you're getting are not a fluke or a mirage—this is a method of systematic weight loss that insists that you eat like *you*. It's the anti-diet that has no part of calorie deprivation or fitting into someone else's rigid program. Some people on The Plan like to start with a cleanse day on Monday; they feel it helps them make better choices for the whole week. Others dine out two or three times a week and stay strictly on The Plan the rest of the week. Play around with it and you will find your own balance. Remember that the scale is your best friend. Or, as one of my clients put it, the scale is her doctor, because it advises her daily on the best choices to make.

Frequently Asked Questions for Phase Three

Should I continue taking the liver detox supplement or tonic?

You certainly can, yes. The liver is responsible for over five hundred functions, remember, and it's good to give it some extra support. If you drink alcohol often, take regular medications, or are exposed to chemicals often, I would recommend taking the liver detox supplement on a regular basis. Just take a week or two off every couple of months to allow your body to reset itself.

Do I need to continue avoiding water after 7:30 p.m.?

If you are just having a friendly day when you know you lose weight, then no, it doesn't matter if you drink past 7:30 p.m. But if you are testing a new food, then you do want to stop at least three hours before bedtime so it doesn't confuse the data.

Do I need to continue eating the same amounts of fat as I have been on The Plan?

Yes, yes, yes. For all the reasons we've talked about, fat is essential not just for cellular health, brain functioning, and satiety, but for weight loss. So drizzle on the olive oil, slather on the butter, and enjoy!

How can I work The Plan into my family life?

After Day Three, I find that almost everyone's family is on board, because the foods you eat on The Plan are ones you normally eat every day. If your family is filled with pasta lovers and pasta doesn't work for you, just make the main Plan-friendly course for the whole family and cook up an extra side of pasta for them! This is all about eating normally and choosing the proteins, vegetables, and grains that work for you. It's important to remember if you have kids that they will inherit many of your food sensitivities, so you are actually doing them a favor by cutting out your reactive foods.

Does smoking contribute to inflammation?

It is pretty widely accepted that anything ingested or inhaled, such as cigarette smoke, that contains high heat will trigger inflammation, including barbecued meat and smoke.

What if I stop doing The Plan and want to restart?

The Plan is always here for you as a resource. If you do veer away from eating according to The Plan, you can start again at any time. In fact, I actually recommend redoing the twenty days every six months or so, just to see what, if anything, has changed in your chemistry.

Just about everyone asks how often they can redo the cleanse (yes, it's true: the thing people originally fear the most is what they want to come back to!). I recommend doing the full three days once every seasonal change.

It's interesting to note that your body's response each time might be different. And doing The Plan certainly will get progressively easier! If you did The Plan the first time around and were in poor health, when you redo it, your weight loss may be greater. I had one client who began The Plan suffering from debilitating arthritis. Over the course of twenty days, her arthritic symptoms were greatly relieved, and she lost eight pounds. Three months later, when she redid her twenty days, she began already free of arthritic pain (ie, not in a state of inflammation). This time, she lost eight pounds *in one week!*

Michael, 55

In twenty days on The Plan, I lost fifteen pounds, and my cholesterol dropped from 250 to 197! I feel great and I am continuing to maintain my weight loss three months later. My overall eating patterns have changed to reflect the guidelines of The Plan, and I can quickly recover when I make other choices. The opportunity to enjoy tasty new foods, have some red wine and dark chocolate, and see immediate results helped me stay committed. My wife was following The Plan at the same time, which was an enormous help.

Traveling on The Plan

Most everyone can lose weight if they stay home and cook every meal in their kitchen, strictly adhering to their friendly foods. But that is no way to live! One of the most gratifying things for me has been to see so many of my clients get the joy surrounding food back in their lives, and being able to travel is a huge part of that.

A sixty-seven-year-old client emailed me recently to touch base. She had lost fifty pounds in five months and was now off Lipitor, with a healthy cholesterol level of 147. But what she really wanted to thank me for was that she'd finally lost her fear of gaining weight while traveling! She and her husband had just come back from a two-week trip to Italy, eating every meal at restaurants, and she'd gained only .8 pound. How was that possible? Easy. She just stuck with the foods she knew worked for her when she could, didn't stress about the rest, and relaxed and enjoyed herself.

Guidelines for Traveling on The Plan

- Be sure to hydrate properly. This is especially important if you will be eating many restaurant meals.
- Incorporate as many of your friendly foods as possible.
- Stick to half portions of any foods that you haven't tested or that you know are reactive for you and surround them with friendly foods.
- Moderate any excess sodium you might be consuming by including foods high in potassium (salt-free potato chips and guacamole, for example).
- If wine is something you enjoy, have a glass or two of red—it acts as a diuretic to flush out excess sodium and aids digestion.
- Relax and enjoy. Really. I mean it. Remember the joy factor? This is what life is all about. And if you need a little extra motivation, think of it this way: being stressed out over not following The Plan perfectly only increases the cortisol in your system, which promotes weight gain. So if you want to maintain your glowing health and weight loss, joy is a must!

Special Occasions

By now I think you know what I'm going to say here. Having a good time is crucial for our well-being and for our health, so please, have fun!

Every year around the holidays, I start getting questions about how to handle big events like Thanksgiving dinner and parties. And my answer is always the same: follow the general guidelines for when you're dining out or traveling, have a little bit of whatever you love, and enjoy.

If you're going to a big family gathering, you can always bring a dish that works for you. Make that your main course and enjoy bites of everything else. Yes, even that food that is high reactive—the new stimulus might prove out better than you think! I had one client who had been eating perfectly on The Plan. Then she went to a family dinner and couldn't resist the mac and cheese and ice cream. She was shocked that she went down .6 pound the next day!

My only caveat here is that I'd say to avoid foods that don't work for you health-wise. We *all* indulge occasionally—and we should, as long as we're not impairing our health. Remember that if you gain, the weight will come off after you get back on your Plan. You always have the option to return to a few winning days that have worked for you in the past to get your body right back on track.

If you're on the holiday merry-go-round of party after party and you're frankly dreading having to eat one more plate of bad food (how many pigs in a blanket can you really stand, after all?), then the best bet is to eat Plan friendly beforehand and just nibble on appetizers when you get to the party. You can also try switching up your lunch and dinner that day so you have a hearty lunch and don't enter the party starving. We generally make poor choices when we are hungry and have had a glass of wine!

What About Cocktails?

Can you drink alcohol on The Plan? Yes, of course! You already know about red wine, which is low reactive. If you enjoy white wine, liquor, or any other kind of cocktail, I encourage you to test it. And if you can't test it before you head out to a special occasion, go ahead and indulge—you know exactly what to do the next day if the scale ticks upward.

Frankly, alcohol is usually not a problem unless you have beer or champagne or mix soda with hard alcohol (carbonation impairs digestion). Beer is high in yeast, which so many people have underlying issues with. And between the carbonation, acidic white wine, and added sugars, which can aggravate yeast, I call champagne the devil in a red dress...with high heels. I'm not telling you not to have any of these things if you enjoy them. Just know the reactivity potential, be proactive by taking a probiotic, and plan for a friendly day the next day or two.

The good news is that many cocktails, such as margaritas or cosmopolitans, are Plan friendly if they are made with fresh lime juice. Fresh lemon and lime help your liver process the alcohol. Remember that whenever we lighten the load on our vital organs, we are always rewarded with better weight loss.

Exercise on The Plan

I'm a huge fan of exercise and its health benefits. What I'm not a fan of is taking time away from your friends and family to spend hours and hours at it, thinking you need to exercise like crazy to lose weight and all the while creating stress on your body. When it comes to exercise, more does not necessarily mean better. For weight loss, it is ideal to limit your workouts to four times a week; more than that and we've seen weight loss stall. The same goes for intensity: extreme workouts like boot camps tend to have the opposite effect on weight loss from what people intend.

Finding what form, duration, and intensity are best for your body is really important, and I encourage you to take the time to find out what works best for you. Testing different kinds and durations of exercise is exactly the same as testing a new food: you take any friendly day you've had and replicate it, inserting the exercise as the variable. You'll know if you've pushed yourself too far if you see your weight loss stall and all the other factors for the prior day were on the mark (foods, water intake, sodium levels, sleep, and stress levels, etc.).

In the Five-Day Self-Test in Part Five, you'll see that the exercise test is programmed on Day Twenty-Four (that is, Day Four of the Self-Test), but you can choose to do it at any point after your twenty days that works best for you. As with any test, if your body has a reactive response, be sure to take a few rest days after that to give your system a chance to recover and reset before resuming testing.

The types of exercise we've found to be most problematic for weight loss are boot camp, spinning, heavy interval training, CrossFit and Bikram yoga. This doesn't mean those won't work for you; I just don't want you putting undue stress on your body, so please make sure to test your exercise. We have had clients who lost weight when they did a thirty-minute run but gained when they increased their running time to more than an hour. I had one client who refused to believe that his fifty-plus-mile bike rides were triggering his auto-immune disease and his consistent two-pound weight gain after each ride. Don't assume that harder and faster are better. Find *your* balance.

The Evolution of Reactivity

Your body is constantly changing, and so is your chemistry. Just as you may have hit some inflammatory speed bumps in your life up until now (the most common ones are ages thirty-five, forty-two, and fifty, or at perimenopause, and at times of ill health or extreme stress), there may be others on the road ahead. So how do you know when your chemistry is shifting and when a friendly food in your rotation might be drifting to the wrong side of the reactivity tracks?

Your scale.

Simply use your scale to gauge when you might need to stop or slow down on a certain food. If you start consistently gaining or stabilizing on foods that have normally worked for you, it might be a sign that your chemistry is changing. You know how to collect the data. Pay attention to what you're eating on the days when you're stabilizing or gaining and you'll find the common denominator so you can formally retest it.

I'm my own best example of this. I used to be able to eat steak and lose half a pound consistently. I cooked up a delicious steak every Sunday night for years and did great. Then age forty-two rolled around, and my migraines start kicking up again. I'd been easily moderating those migraines for almost thirty years with nutrition and herbs, so naturally I was very concerned and looked to my scale for clues.

I started noticing that I was up half a pound every Monday morning. At first I blamed the fun stuff—too much chocolate or bread—but I quickly realized that steak was the constant. I cut out the steak, and my migraines disappeared, along with the Monday-morning weight bump. The weight that would have slowly started to creep on, which hits most of us in our forties, was stopped in its tracks. My chemistry had changed; I'd hit an inflammatory speed bump and my body had become sensitive to steak.

I know how The Plan works, and I know that if you cut out a reactive food, there's a good chance your body will heal. So I tested myself on steak again six months later. This time I stabilized. I didn't experience any migraines, which was great, but my response in weight was not what it had been, so I continued to leave steak out of my menu plans. I tested it again a few times over the next few years and got the same results. Three years later, I tested steak and lost a pound, no migraines. Now I have steak every once in a while and thoroughly enjoy it.

Knowing that steak is a potentially inflammatory food for me, how do I know when to stop eating it? My scale. As soon as I start stabilizing or gaining after I eat steak, that's my sign that I need to cut back.

Living The Plan goes beyond just reaching your goal weight and state of health; it's a lifelong relationship you're building with your body so that you'll know which foods allow it to run at optimal levels. Your body is talking to you all the time via the numbers on the scale, health symptoms, or mood. If you pay attention to your body's signals, it really will tell you everything you need to know.

Yvonne, 43

As a busy executive working in government and politics, giving attention to my well-being and to healthy eating was never a priority. I started The Plan when iron-deficiency anemia stopped me in my tracks. My blood count was 10 and I was seriously ill. After five months on The Plan, my count was 34 and I had lost twenty-five pounds. Almost a year later I'm a healthy size four and feel better than ever. The Plan transformed my life and helped me make health my top priority.

The Plan for Lifelong Health

Perhaps you picked up this book because you'd tried every diet out there and still couldn't lose weight…or had a chronic disease or ailment that you couldn't seem to get under control…or because your body's dynamic was changing and you couldn't quite figure out its new rules. Whatever your reason, it's been my joy and honor to help give you your individual road map to lifelong health and weight management.

Will you have ups and downs in the future? Absolutely. That's the nature of our biology. But those ups and downs will never again tyrannize you, because you're in control. *You* are the boss of you, and you have the data squarely in your possession that makes you the ultimate expert on your own body. Remember, you can always lose weight and be healthy; you just need to plug in the data that tells you how your body works. Your body is constantly communicating to you what does and doesn't work for it through weight, mood, and health—all you have to do is listen.

The Plan is always here for you, now and in the future, as a resource and guide. And for even more support, please join The Plan community at www.theplan.com, to hear from thousands of others just like you who have discovered what it truly means to eat, live, and be healthy.

Part Four

THE PLAN RECIPES

This collection of recipes has been created and compiled by me, my staff of nutritionists, and Plan followers around the country. For easy reference, I've divided it into two sections. The first section contains the recipes you'll need to have on hand to follow the prescribed menu plans for Days One through Twenty. The second section contains recipes you can use as you begin testing and experimenting on your own.

Recipes for Days One through Twenty

BREAKFAST

FLAX GRANOLA

Making your own flax granola is very easy. You can double the amounts of ingredients if you wish, to have more granola on hand.

1 cup whole flaxseeds
½ cup water
Cinnamon, nutmeg, cloves to taste
Raisins, almonds, walnuts, dried cranberries, etc., to taste (please be sure to include only nuts you have tested)
Optional: vanilla extract

Mix flaxseeds with water seasoned with cinnamon (and other spices if desired); refrigerate overnight. Spread in a thin layer on a baking sheet and bake at 275 °F for 50 minutes to 1 hour, turning several times to dry out. Optional: add raisins, nuts, and other dried fruits of choice in the last 10 minutes.

Makes 2 to 3 servings.

SMOOTHIE

Rice Dream or Silk coconut milk
1 sun-ripened pear (most pears you buy in the supermarket are unripe; if you put them in the sun they will ripen in a day)
½ cup berries
¼ avocado
Ice
2–4 tablespoons chia seeds
Optional: 1 tsp honey or agave nectar
Optional: vanilla extract or cinnamon

Fill blender with Rice Dream or Silk coconut milk to 16 or 20 oz and add pear, berries, avocado, ice (ice is not recommended if you have thyroid dysfunction), chia seeds, and any optional ingredients desired. Blend until smooth.

Makes 1 serving.

Sauces and Toppings

INDIAN SPICE RUB

6 tbsp salt-free curry powder
1 to 2 tbsp brown sugar
¼ tsp sea salt
1 tbsp crushed red pepper or cayenne
1 tbsp ground cumin
1 tbsp ground coriander
1 tbsp turmeric
1 tbsp cinnamon
1 tbsp ground ginger

Combine curry powder, brown sugar, and sea salt. Add remaining spices, adjusting to taste. Store in airtight container for up to 6 months.

Makes 6 to 8 servings.

LEMON GARLIC SAUCE

15 cloves of garlic, peeled (can buy prepared in stores)
4 tbsp extra virgin olive oil
4 tbsp fresh lemon juice
Sea salt to taste
Freshly ground black pepper to taste

Brush each clove of garlic with olive oil and bake at 400 °F for 40 minutes. Let cool for 10 minutes. Add remaining ingredients and mash, or blend in food processor.

Makes 4 servings.

Herbs to Enhance Digestion and Decrease E. Coli Poisoning

Herbs and spices like oregano, thyme, cinnamon, and cloves do more than add pleasing flavors and aromas. The compounds extracted from the oils of these plants pack a powerful antimicrobial punch—strong enough to help quell such food-borne pathogens as E. coli.

All the herbs and spices we use in The Plan are noted for their antibiotic, antimicrobial, and digestive properties: turmeric, cinnamon, cumin, black pepper, rosemary, garlic, onion, mint, ginger, cloves, etc. So please feel free to include liberally as you cut down on your sodium and enjoy the health benefits!

Growing your own herbs (yes, city dwellers can do it, too!) provides a huge, flavorful treat and makes every meal seem special. When herbs start to flower, use the blossoms as beautiful dressings for your meal.

MANGO SALSA

1 whole mango, chopped
Juice of 1 lime
Optional: ½ small raw red onion
½ roasted jalapeño, minced (or a whole jalapeño for extra spice; to
    roast, lay on open flame until skin starts to blacken) or 1 tablespoon
    of Sriracha sauce

Combine all ingredients and spoon on top of fish or chicken. Serving
size is 2 to 3 tbsp.

Makes 6 to 8 servings.

ORANGE (OR LEMON, OR LIME) OIL

One medium-sized orange (preferably organic, as pesticides cling to the
    natural oils present in citrus skin)
½ cup extra virgin olive oil

Thoroughly wash the rind with soap. Zest the full orange (or lemon
or lime, if you prefer to make Lemon Oil or Lime Oil) and soak in
olive oil. If you prefer a more intensely flavored oil, use two pieces of
citrus. Drizzle the oil on steamed vegetables or broiled fish, or use it
to make a flavorful vinaigrette.

Health Benefits of Citrus Zest Oil

Citrus peels pack a powerful health punch. The oils in the peels of
lemons, oranges, limes, and tangerines contain large amounts of lim-
onene, which encourages the body's detoxification system, enhances
antioxidant activity, and helps fight cancer. Studies have shown that
consuming as little as half a tablespoon of lemon peel a week has
decreased chances of getting skin cancer by 50 percent!

Orange peel contains hesperidin, which reduces the risk of heart disease by lowering LDL cholesterol and triglycerides and helps regulate blood pressure. Research has also shown a correlation between increased use of hesperidin and decreased risk of breast cancer.

Additionally, the pectin in orange and lemon peel acts as a prebiotic. Prebiotics help to encourage the natural growth of probiotic activity, which encourages digestive health and proper immune functioning.

SPICY APRICOT GLAZE

½ cup apricot jam
¼ to ½ cup water
1 tbsp chipotles in adobo sauce or 2 tsp smoked chipotle powder
   (optional: substitute Sriracha)

Combine all ingredients and mix until smooth.

Makes 12 to 16 servings.

SPICY COCO SAUCE

This sauce is legendary among Plan followers. It's so delicious that I've had clients say they would eat pretty much anything if it had Spicy Coco Sauce on it!

1 large onion, chopped
3 to 4 cloves garlic, chopped
Ginger, cinnamon, cumin, turmeric, freshly ground black pepper,
   cayenne (all to taste)
1 can coconut milk (please do not use low-fat)
½ tsp sea salt
1 heaping tbsp brown sugar

Sauté onion, garlic, and spices in coconut milk. Add salt and brown sugar and reduce for 20 minutes. Sauce will hold for 5 days refrigerated, or you can freeze it. Portion size is ⅛ cup per serving.

Makes 4 servings.

Soup, Salads, and Snacks

BEET AND CARROT SALAD

4 to 5 whole carrots
1 small beet
Peel carrots and beet. Grate all and mix together in one bowl.

Makes 4 servings.

CARROT GINGER SOUP (ALTERNATE RECIPE ON PAGE 295)

Carrot Ginger is an excellent anti-inflammatory soup. If you experience reactivity, you can always add some of this soup to your lunch to soothe your digestive system.

1½ lb carrots
1 zucchini
1 onion
2 to 3 cloves garlic
Raw ginger, peeled and minced, to taste
Cinnamon, cumin, onion powder to taste
Freshly ground black pepper to taste
1 quart water

Chop vegetables and simmer with spices in water (for thicker soup, use ½ quart of water) until soft. Puree in blender or food processor.

Makes 6 to 8 servings.

SAUTÉED KALE WITH VEGETABLES

5 to 6 cups chopped kale
4 shiitake mushrooms, chopped
2 tbsp extra virgin olive oil
Herbs of your choice

Sauté kale and shiitakes in olive oil with herbs of choice. Let cool and add your favorite topping (pumpkin seeds, cheese, avocado, almond slivers, etc.), or mix in other vegetables to test.

Makes 2 servings.

KALE, CHICKPEA, AND GOAT CHEESE SALAD

1 bunch kale
2 tbsp extra virgin olive oil
½ cup low-sodium chickpeas
½ apple, chopped
2 ounces goat or sheep's milk cheese
Lime Agave Vinaigrette (page 192)

Sauté kale in extra virgin olive oil for 1 to 2 minutes. Add chickpeas. Finish with apple, cheese, and Lime Agave Vinaigrette. Once you have tested mustard, you can substitute Mustard Vinaigrette (page 193) for the Lime Agave, if you prefer.

Makes 2 to 3 servings.

ROASTED SQUASH, KALE, AND MANCHEGO SALAD

1 delicata or butternut squash, cut into 1-inch chunks
1 bunch kale
3 shiitake mushrooms, slivered
2 tablespoons extra virgin olive oil
2 to 3 oz Manchego
Optional: cremini mushrooms (moderate reactivity)
Optional: if tested, add walnuts or steamed green beans
Dressing of choice

Roast squash at 425 °F for 30 minutes or steam for 5 to 6 minutes. Sauté kale and shiitakes in extra virgin olive oil for 2 to 3 minutes and add squash. Top with grated Manchego. Add optional ingredients, if using, and top with dressing.

Makes 4 servings.

SPICY CHICKPEA SPINACH SALAD

Turmeric, ginger, cinnamon, cayenne, all to taste
3 to 4 cloves garlic, chopped
1 medium onion, chopped
Sea salt
1 15-ounce can low-sodium chickpeas
4 to 6 cups organic baby spinach (please omit spinach and replace with
    mixed greens if you have thyroid dysfunction)
¼ cup grated carrot
¼ cup cup pumpkin seeds

Sauté turmeric, ginger, cinnamon, cayenne, garlic, and onion with dash of salt. Simmer for 3 minutes and add chickpeas. Simmer for another 10 minutes, stirring frequently. Add spinach. Allow spinach to wilt (this enhances the bioavailability of the iron in the spinach) and finish with grated carrot and pumpkin seeds.

Makes 2 to 4 servings.

SPICY VEGETARIAN SOUP

1 onion, chopped
4 cloves garlic, chopped
1 tbsp poultry seasoning
1 tbsp cumin
2 tbsp Sriracha
2 tsp peeled and grated ginger
1 to 2 tsp honey
1 quart water
1 quart low-sodium vegetable broth
1 bunch kale
1 butternut squash, chopped
3 zucchini, chopped
3 carrots, chopped
1 head broccoli, chopped
1 (15-ounce) can of chick peas or ¾ cup cooked chick peas
1 bay leaf
As you discover your friendly vegetables, add them to this basic soup

Sauté onion, garlic, poultry seasoning, cumin, Sriracha, and honey. Add water, vegetable broth, and vegetables and simmer for 30 minutes; add bay leaf 5 minutes before end of cooking and remove before eating. You can either enjoy this soup as is or, if you prefer, puree it.

Makes 4 to 6 servings.

THE PLAN CHOPPED SALAD

5 to 6 cups baby romaine lettuce, chopped
1 large zucchini, diced
1 large carrot, diced
1 apple, chopped
½ avocado
Handful of sunflower seeds
Dill to taste
Optional: red onion, diced

Combine romaine, zucchini, and carrot. Add apple, avocado, sunflower seeds, cilantro, and onion, if desired, and serve with vinaigrette of choice.

Makes 4 servings.

HOMEMADE HUMMUS

2 cups drained well-cooked or low-sodium canned chickpeas, liquid reserved
¼ cup extra virgin olive oil, plus more for drizzling
2 cloves garlic, peeled
Sea salt and freshly ground black pepper to taste
1 tbsp ground cumin, or to taste, plus a sprinkling for garnish
Juice of 1 lemon
Chopped fresh parsley leaves for garnish

Put everything except parsley in food processor and begin to process; add chickpea liquid or water as needed to produce a smooth puree.

Taste and adjust seasonings (you may want to add more lemon juice). Serve drizzled with olive oil and sprinkled with a bit more cumin and some parsley.

Makes 8 to 10 servings.

BUTTERNUT SQUASH SOUP

1 large butternut or delicata squash
2 zucchini
1 large onion
1 tbsp fresh ginger
1 quart water
Cinnamon, black pepper, onion powder, all to taste

Chop vegetables and ginger, and simmer with spices in water (for thicker soup, use ½ quart of water) until soft. Puree in blender or food processor.

Makes 2 to 4 servings.

CHOCOLATE-COVERED PEAR SLICES

2 oz dark chocolate
3 tbsp chia seeds
1 pear cut into 6 to 8 slices

Melt chocolate in microwave. Add chia seeds and drizzle over pear slices. Place on wax paper and let cool.

Makes 3 to 4 servings.

DINNER

CHICKEN WITH ITALIAN HERBS AND ORANGE ZEST

1 orange
Dried Italian herbs
2 portions chicken breasts (one portion is 4 to 6 ounces for women and 6 to 8 ounces for men)

Wash the orange thoroughly and grate the skin until you have 2 tablespoons' worth of orange zest. Set aside. Liberally sprinkle Italian herbs on chicken so each breast is covered. Add orange zest and bake at 350 °F for 20 to 30 minutes, depending on the thickness of the breasts.

Makes 2 servings.

VEGETABLE TIMBALE

1 large zucchini
1 red onion
½ bunch Swiss chard (use kale if you have thyroid dysfunction)
4 to 6 oz soft goat cheese, crumbled
1½ large carrots
8 shiitake mushrooms
2 oz Parmesan or Manchego, grated

Preheat oven to 400 °F. Use a mandoline or slice vegetables as thinly as you can. Create layers as for lasagna, laying vegetables and goat cheese in a 9-inch baking dish (does not need to be oiled): zucchini, onion, Swiss chard, goat cheese, carrots, shiitakes, etc., and top with Parmesan or Manchego. Cook for 30 minutes, or until cheese on top is slightly golden.

Makes 6 servings.

HEALTHY CHICKEN PARMESAN

2 portions chicken breast or thighs
2 plum tomatoes
2 tbsp extra virgin olive oil
2 to 3 cloves garlic
⅛ cup fresh basil
Sea salt and freshly ground black pepper to taste
Optional: fresh rosemary and oregano to taste
3 oz fresh unsalted mozzarella or goat Cheddar, grated
1 oz Parmesan

Prepare chicken to your liking (broil, grill, etc.). Dice and sauté tomatoes in olive oil with garlic, basil, salt and pepper, and optional herbs, if desired, for 2 minutes. Place sautéed tomatoes on cooked chicken and top with cheeses. Broil on high for 3 to 4 minutes, or until cheese starts to brown.

Makes 2 servings.

LAMB BURGERS

1 lb ground lamb
1 zucchini, grated
4 to 5 shiitake mushrooms, chopped
Herbs and spices of choice (Italian herb blend, Herbes de Provence, cumin, turmeric, fresh ground pepper, Sriricha, etc.)

Combine all ingredients, form into 4 patties, and pan sear to medium rare, 6 to 8 minutes.

Makes 4 servings.

ROASTED ITALIAN WINTER VEGETABLES

What is better and easier than roasted fall or winter vegetables? Roasting always makes the house nice and toasty warm—yum!

3 large carrots
1 large zucchini
1 head broccoli
1 medium onion
4 to 5 cloves garlic
3 tbsp extra virgin olive oil
Italian herbs, fresh or dried, to taste
Sea salt and freshly ground black pepper to taste

Preheat oven to 375 °F. Chop vegetables and toss with olive oil, herbs, salt, and pepper. If you have time, let mixture stand for 30 minutes before baking for 30 minutes.

Later, once you begin testing on your own, this recipe is great for adding potatoes, Brussels sprouts, or other vegetables you want to test. There is something about the combination of these vegetables that offsets the potential problems of potatoes (weight gain) and Brussels sprouts (higher reactivity and gas).

Makes 4 servings.

DESSERTS

CINNAMON POACHED FRUIT

½ apple or pear
¼ cup water or wine (for stovetop method)
Sprinkle of cinnamon
Optional: fresh whipped cream for topping

Stovetop: Poach fruit in ¼ cup water or wine, add cinnamon, and let simmer for 2 minutes.

Microwave method: Cook apple or pear, sprinkled with cinnamon, microwave on high for 45 seconds.

Makes 1 serving.

Recipes for Testing on Your Own

The recipes in this section have been selected for Phase Three and beyond, to give you some options for testing new foods—and to encourage you to experiment with new ways to enjoy some of your Plan-friendly favorites.

APPLE PANCAKES WITH CINNAMON BUTTER

For pancakes:

2 medium sweet apples (scant 1 lb), peeled, halved, and cored
1 tsp orange zest
1⅔ cups all-purpose flour
2 tbsp (packed) golden brown sugar
2½ tsp baking powder
½ tsp sea salt
¾ cup Silk vanilla coconut milk or Rice Dream
2 large eggs
½ cup (1 stick) unsalted butter, melted, divided

For cinnamon butter:

½ cup (1 stick) unsalted butter, room temperature
½ cup powdered sugar
1 tsp ground cinnamon
½ tsp grated orange peel

For pancakes: Coarsely grate apples into medium bowl. Add zest and toss. In a separate bowl, whisk flour, brown sugar, baking powder, and salt. Make a well in center of dry ingredients. Whisk in coconut milk or Rice Dream, eggs, and ¼ cup melted butter until smooth. Stir in apple mixture. Cover and let batter stand at room temperature at least 30 minutes and up to 1 hour.

Preheat oven to 250 °F. Place baking sheet in oven. Heat large, heavy nonstick griddle or skillet over medium-high heat for 1 minute. Brush with some of remaining melted butter. For each pancake, drop a heaping tbsp of batter onto griddle, spacing pancakes a few inches apart. Cook until golden on bottom and bubbles start to form on surface, about 3 minutes. Turn pancakes over. Cook until golden on bottom, about 2 minutes longer. Transfer pancakes to baking sheet in oven to keep warm. Repeat with remaining batter, brushing griddle with butter before each batch of pancakes.

For cinnamon butter: Using electric mixer, beat all ingredients in small bowl until blended.

Top each pancake with a dollop of cinnamon butter and serve.

Makes 8 to 10 pancakes.

JESSICA'S ZUCCHINI BREAD

(can also be made as muffins)

¼ cup honey
1 egg
¼ cup applesauce
¼ cup butter
2 cups shredded zucchini
2 tsp lemon zest
2 tbsp lemon juice
1½ cups all-purpose flour
½ tsp baking soda
¼ tsp baking powder
1 tsp ground cinnamon

Preheat oven to 325 °F. Grease an 8x4-inch loaf pan.

In a bowl, beat together honey, egg, and applesauce. Add zucchini, lemon zest, and juice. In a separate bowl, sift together flour, baking soda, baking powder, and cinnamon. Stir flour mixture into zucchini mixture until just blended. Pour batter into prepared pan.

Bake 45 minutes, until a knife inserted in center comes out clean. Cool about 10 minutes before turning out onto a wire rack to cool completely.

Makes 8 to 10 servings.

SAUCES AND TOPPINGS

BLUEBERRY BOURBON MARINADE (SPICY)

2 tbsp coconut oil
1 red onion, chopped
Garlic, chopped
Chipotles in adobo sauce or Sriracha to taste
½ cup bourbon
2 cups fresh blueberries
¼ cup homemade tomato sauce from plum tomatoes
¼ cup apple cider vinegar
⅛ cup brown sugar
Cinnamon to taste

Heat oil in a large saucepan over medium heat. Add onion and sauté for 2 to 4 minutes, or until tender and just starting to brown. Add garlic and chipotles or Sriracha and sauté for 3 to 4 minutes. Add bourbon, increase heat to high, and bring to a boil to reduce for approximately 5 minutes (this burns off the alcohol as well). Stir in blueberries, tomato sauce, vinegar, brown sugar, and cinnamon, and simmer for 20 minutes.

Makes 8 to 10 servings

CHIMICHURRI SAUCE

5 cloves garlic
2 tbsp chopped red onion
2 cups fresh parsley or cilantro, firmly packed
¼ cup fresh oregano leaves
½ cup extra virgin olive oil
3 tbsp lime or lemon juice
Sea salt, freshly ground black pepper, and red pepper flakes to taste

Pulse garlic and onion in a food processor until finely chopped. Add parsley or cilantro and oregano, and pulse again briefly, until finely chopped. Transfer mixture to a bowl. Add olive oil and lime or lemon juice and stir. (Adding the liquids outside the food processor gives the chimichurri the correct texture. You don't want the herbs to be completely pureed, just finely chopped.) Season with salt, black pepper, and red pepper flakes to taste. Store in the refrigerator until ready to serve.

Makes 8 to 10 servings

CUBAN MARINADE

2 shallots, chopped
¼ cup coarsely chopped fresh mint
1 tsp freshly grated lemon zest
¼ cup dark rum
½ cup lime juice (Santa Cruz and Whole Foods' 365 brand sell great organic lime juice in glass bottles)
2 to 3 tbsp honey
Dash of sea salt

Combine all ingredients and use as a marinade for your protein of choice.

Makes 6 to 8 servings

FRENCH ROAST BALSAMIC MARINADE

½ cup strong French roast coffee
4 tbsp balsamic vinegar
2 to 3 tbsp dark brown sugar
2 to 3 tbsp extra virgin olive oil
2 to 3 garlic cloves, chopped
¼ tsp sea salt
Freshly ground black pepper to taste

Combine all ingredients and use ½ cup to marinate beef or lamb. Reserve remaining marinade for basting.

Makes 8 servings.

FRUIT SALSA (MEDIUM HOT)

Pineapple, peach, apricot, and mango all lend themselves beautifully to salsa.

Fruit of choice, about 2 cups
1 roasted jalapeño pepper with seeds (2 jalapeños for extra hot; to roast, lay on open flame until skin starts to blacken)
½ small red onion
2 tbsp lime juice
1 tbsp agave nectar
Dash of sea salt
Freshly ground black pepper
¼ tsp allspice or toasted cinnamon

Chop fruit, jalapeño, and onion and combine. Add remaining ingredients.

Makes 8 to 10 servings

HORSERADISH APPLE CRUST FOR FISH

4 tbsp prepared horseradish
½ Granny Smith apple, grated
1 cup bread crumbs (regular or panko)
1 tbsp butter, melted

Combine horseradish, apple, and bread crumbs and pat out excess liquid. Add melted butter and spread mixture on fish fillets. Broil for 8 to 10 minutes, until crust is browned and fish is cooked through.

Makes 4 to 6 servings.

JAMAICAN JERK SEASONING

¼ cup ground allspice

Cinnamon to taste

Freshly grated nutmeg to taste

½ tsp dried thyme

1 bunch scallions, thinly sliced

2 to 3 garlic cloves

2 Scotch bonnet or other chili peppers of choice (optional: Sriracha or chipotles in adobo sauce to taste)

3 tbsp dark rum

Freshly squeezed juice of ½ orange

½ tsp sea salt (do not use salt unless using fresh chili pepper, as Sriracha and chipotles in adobo already contain salt)

Freshly ground black pepper to taste

Stir allspice, cinnamon, nutmeg, and thyme in a small skillet over medium-low heat for 3 minutes to toast. Put in food processor with scallions, garlic, chili peppers, rum, orange juice, salt, and pepper; blend to a smooth paste.

Makes 6 to 8 servings.

JILL'S MONTREAL STEAK SEASONING

1 tbsp coarse sea salt

1 tbsp freshly ground black pepper

1 tbsp dehydrated onion

½ tbsp dehydrated garlic

½ tbsp crushed red pepper

½ tbsp dried thyme

½ tbsp dried rosemary

½ tbsp dried fennel

Combine ingredients and store in a shaker. Shake or rub 1 tbsp seasoning onto steaks, pork chops, or hamburgers before grilling.

Makes 5 servings.

LEMON ZEST VINAIGRETTE

2 medium-sized lemons or 1 small orange
½ cup extra virgin olive oil
¼ cup Balsamic vinegar
1 to 2 garlic cloves, mashed
Herbs of choice (I like Herbes de Provence in this recipe)

Zest lemons or orange and let steep in oil for at least 1 full day, but preferably 4 to 5 days, before making vinaigrette. Use 2 parts steeped olive oil to 1 part balsamic vinegar and 1 to 2 mashed garlic cloves; add herbs of choice. Store in a closed container in the refrigerator for up to 1 week.

Makes 8 servings.

LIME AGAVE VINAIGRETTE

¼ cup freshly squeezed lime juice
¼ cup extra virgin olive oil
⅛ cup water
1 tbsp Herbes de Provence
1 tbsp agave nectar
Optional: 1 clove garlic, crushed

Combine all ingredients in a bowl and mix together well. Store in a closed container in the refrigerator for up to 1 week.

Makes 6 to 8 servings.

LINDSEY'S FAJITA MARINADE

3 tbsp olive oil
Juice of 1 lime
2 cloves garlic, minced or grated
1-inch piece of fresh ginger, minced or grated
1 tsp lemon zest
2 tsp turmeric
½ tsp cumin
Optional: pinch of chili flakes
¼ tsp sea salt

Combine all ingredients and use as a marinade for your protein of choice.

Makes 4 to 6 servings.

MUSTARD VINAIGRETTE

1 clove garlic, smashed
2 tbsp balsamic vinegar (or apple cider vinegar, which has a long history of relieving arthritic pain)
1 tsp Dijon mustard
5 to 6 tbsp extra virgin olive oil
Dried herbs (parsley, thyme)
Dash of onion powder
Freshly ground black pepper

Combine all ingredients and use as a dressing on your favorite salad. Store in a closed container in the refrigerator for up to 1 week.

Makes 8 servings.

AMY'S SUNFLOWER BUTTER SALAD DRESSING

1 large garlic clove, crushed
4 tbsp extra virgin olive oil
1 to 2 tbsp sunflower butter
2 tbsp apple cider vinegar
1 to 2 tsp honey
Sea salt and freshly ground black pepper to taste

Whisk garlic into olive oil. Add sunflower butter, vinegar, and honey and stir. Add salt and pepper to taste. Use as a dressing on your favorite salad. Store in a closed container in the refrigerator for up to 1 week.

Makes 4 to 6 servings.

MARINADE FOR FISH, CHICKEN, OR PORK

(moderate to high reactivity)

½ cup orange juice
½ cup fresh basil or 1 tbsp dried basil
2 cloves garlic
1 tbsp brown sugar
Optional: cayenne to taste

Combine all ingredients and marinate protein for ½ hour. Sauté protein and add ½ of marinade mixture to pan for last 5 to 7 minutes of cooking time.

Makes 4 servings.

OJ-GINGER DRESSING

(moderate to high reactivity)

2 cups orange juice
3 tbsp grated fresh ginger
½ tsp agave

Add ginger to orange juice in saucepan and heat for about 20 minutes, or until orange juice is reduced by ½, then add agave and simmer 1 minute more. This dressing is great served over vegetables, baked chicken, or broiled fish. Store in a closed container in the refrigerator for up to 1 week.

Makes 16 servings.

SATE SAUCE

½ cup water
½ cup coconut milk
2 cloves garlic, minced
2 tbsp Sriracha sauce, or to taste
4 tbsp crunchy peanut butter or raw almond butter
1 tsp brown sugar

Combine water, coconut milk, garlic, and Sriracha sauce in pan and simmer. Add peanut butter and brown sugar and stir until well combined. This can be kept in the fridge for up to one week.

Makes 6 to 8 servings.

SEASONED NUTS

1 to 2 tbsp cinnamon, or to taste
Any digestive spices you like (ginger, etc.)
2 tbsp extra virgin olive oil
1 cup raw nuts of choice
⅛ cup maple syrup

Sauté cinnamon (and other spices of your choice) in olive oil. Add walnuts and stir for 1 minute, then add maple syrup to coat. Let cool in refrigerator. Holds for 2 weeks in an airtight container.

Makes 8 servings.

SHEEP'S MILK YOGURT DRESSING

(moderate reactivity)

1 cup sheep's milk yogurt
1 small Kirby cucumber, peeled and diced
½ cup fresh dill, chopped

Combine all ingredients; serve chilled. Store in a closed container in the refrigerator for up to 1 week.

Makes 16 servings.

SPICY PEANUT SAUCE

⅓ cup peanut butter, softened
4 tbsp water
3 to 4 tbsp lime juice
1 tbsp minced fresh ginger
1 clove garlic, minced
1 tbsp Sriracha, or to taste
Optional: 1 tbsp agave nectar

Whisk together all ingredients in a small bowl. If needed, you can microwave the peanut butter for a few seconds first to soften it up. Works great as a dip for crudité, as a salad dressing, or on chicken.

Makes 8 to 10 servings.

SALADS, SNACKS, AND SOUPS

APPLE CUMIN CHIPS

2 tsp cumin
Dash of sea salt
Freshly ground black pepper to taste
2 medium Granny Smith apples

Preheat oven to 200 °F. Combine cumin, salt, and pepper. Place ½ of cumin mixture on parchment paper or nonstick pan. Use a mandoline to cut apples into very thin slices, approximately ⅛ of an inch. Place on cumin mixture on prepared pan; sprinkle remaining cumin mixture over. Bake 90 minutes, until crisp. Immediately peel slices off pan and let cool. Slices keep for 1 week in an airtight container. Makes a great Plan-friendly snack with hummus or nut butter!

Makes 4 servings.

BEET "CARPACCIO"

2 to 3 medium-sized beets
⅛ cup lemon juice
¼ cup extra virgin olive oil
Dash of sea salt
2 to 3 tbsp chopped dill or herb of choice
1 to 2 cloves garlic

Slice beets on a mandoline. Combine all other ingredients and let beets marinate 24 hours. Serve with a nice spicy green like watercress or arugula. The leftover marinade makes an excellent vinaigrette.

Makes 6 to 8 servings.

AVOCADO–GOAT CHEESE SALAD WITH LIME DRESSING

1½ cups matchstick-sized strips peeled jicama (or zucchini if jicama is not available)
¼ cup extra virgin olive oil
3 tbsp fresh lime juice
5-oz package mixed greens
Sea salt and freshly ground black pepper to taste
1 large avocado, peeled, pitted, sliced
5-oz package soft fresh goat cheese

Toss first 4 ingredients in a large bowl. Sprinkle with salt and pepper. Add avocado and goat cheese; toss gently.

Makes 4 servings.

BASMATI RICE SALAD

1 diced cucumber
3 cups diced arugula or spinach
2 grated carrots
Mint or parsley to taste
1 small onion, chopped
1 yellow zucchini, chopped
3 to 4 shiitake mushrooms, chopped
Herbs and spices of choice
1 cup cooked basmati rice
Optional: raisins, sunflower seeds, pumpkin seeds

Combine cucumber, arugula or spinach, carrots, and mint or parsley and set aside. Sauté onion, zucchini, and mushrooms with herbs and spices and add to salad mixture, letting heat of cooked vegetables slightly wilt arugula or spinach. (This will decrease the chance of negatively affecting thyroid if there is thyroid dysfunction.) Combine all ingredients with cooked rice. Optional: add raisins for iron, sunflower seeds for calcium, and pumpkin seeds for immune and/or prostate health.

Makes 2 to 4 servings.

CHICKEN ESCAROLE ONION SOUP

6 boneless chicken thighs, cut into quarters
2 stalks celery, sliced into 2-inch pieces (can include leaves for extra flavor)
2 whole carrots, coarsely chopped
2 large onions, chopped
1 parsnip, coarsely chopped
2 tbsp chopped fresh dill
2 tbsp chopped fresh parsley
¼ tsp sea salt
Freshly ground black pepper
1 lb escarole, chopped

Fill a large pot with 4 quarts water; place over high heat and bring to a boil. Add chicken and return to boil, skimming off any foam that accumulates on top. Reduce heat to low and continue cooking, uncovered, for 2 hours.

Add celery, carrots, onions, parsnip, dill, and parsley. Continue cooking slowly, uncovered, for 1 hour.

Set a strainer over a large bowl and strain soup; discard solids. Season with salt and pepper. Refrigerate, covered, overnight.

Remove layer of fat that has formed on soup and discard. Place soup in a large saucepan and bring to a boil. Just before serving, add escarole and cook until just tender, about 3 minutes.

Makes 8 to 10 servings.

DANDELION SALAD WITH LEMON VINAIGRETTE

For salad:
½ bunch dandelion greens
1 oz Manchego, grated
Sunflower seeds
1 apple, chopped

For lemon vinaigrette:
1½ tsp finely grated orange zest
Freshly squeezed juice of 1 lemon
Pinch of sea salt
Freshly ground black pepper
6 tbsp extra virgin olive oil

Mix salad ingredients in a bowl. Combine vinaigrette ingredients and toss with salad to coat.

Makes 2 to 3 servings.

FRIED RED POTATO WITH GREENS

1 small red potato
Optional: 4 to 5 shiitake mushrooms
2 tbsp extra virgin olive oil
1 bunch kale or 8 cups mixed greens
2 oz Parmesan cheese, shaved
Freshly ground black pepper

Slice red potato into thin slices and lightly fry in olive oil (with shiitakes if desired) until they are soft to the touch with a fork. Toss with mixed greens or steamed kale, Parmesan cheese shavings, and pepper.

Makes 4 servings.

JESSICA'S AVOCADO CHICKEN SALAD

1 chicken breast or thigh, cooked and shredded
½ avocado
1 tsp mayonnaise
1 green onion, sliced
Dill, to taste
Lime juice, to taste
Sea salt and freshly ground black pepper to taste

Combine all ingredients in a bowl.

Makes 2 servings.

KAFAYAT'S INDONESIAN CHICKEN SOUP

1 free-range chicken, about 3 lb, quartered
2 stalks fresh lemongrass, bruised with the handle of a heavy knife and
 tied in a knot
Optional: 6 kaffir lime leaves, fresh or frozen
½ tsp sea salt
2 quarts water
1 tsp black peppercorns
1½ tbsp coriander seeds
2 tsp cumin seeds
5 shallots, peeled and halved
3 cloves garlic, peeled
1½ tsp turmeric
2 tbsp finely minced fresh ginger
2 tbsp extra virgin olive oil
1 tbsp fresh lime juice
Optional: 4 oz glass noodles or thin dried rice noodles
2 tbsp chopped cilantro
Optional: 2 shallots, thinly sliced and fried in vegetable oil until brown
Quartered limes and chili flakes

Place chicken in a medium pot with lemongrass, lime leaves (if using), salt, and water. Bring to a boil over high heat. Skim off any foam and reduce heat to a simmer. Cover and simmer until chicken is tender, about 45 minutes, skimming as needed to make a clear broth. Remove chicken pieces from broth and set aside. Remove and discard lemongrass and lime leaves; reserve stock in pot. When chicken is cool enough to handle, discard skin and bones and shred meat into bite-sized pieces.

Meanwhile, combine peppercorns, coriander seeds, and cumin seeds in a small food processor. Pulse until ground. Add shallots, garlic, turmeric, and ginger, and pulse to a thick paste. (Add a little water if needed.) Heat oil in a medium saucepan over high heat. When very hot, add spice paste and cook, stirring, until paste is cooked and beginning to separate from oil, about 5 minutes.

Add cooked spice paste and chicken to stock. Bring to a simmer and cook 10 minutes. Turn off heat and stir in lime juice. Add additional salt salt to taste.

If desired, cook noodles according to package directions. To serve, divide noodles among 4 large soup bowls. Ladle soup on top and sprinkle with cilantro, and fried shallots, if using. Pass quartered limes and chili flakes at the table.

Makes 4 servings.

KALE AND BLACK-EYED PEA SOUP

2 cups water
2 cups low-sodium chicken stock
3 cups dried black-eyed peas
1 medium onion, chopped
4 to 5 carrots
1 bay leaf
6 cups chopped kale

Bring water and chicken stock to a boil. Add black-eyed peas (no need to soak first), onion, carrots, bay leaf, and kale. Let simmer for 45 minutes and remove bay leaf.

Makes 6 to 8 servings.

KAVEETA'S CHOPPED SALAD

3 medium zucchini, sliced lengthwise ⅓ inch thick
1 bunch scallions, white and light green parts only
2 chicken breasts (6 oz each)
3 tbsp extra virgin olive oil
Coarse sea salt
1 large avocado
2 heads butter lettuce, leaves separated, cut into thick strips
⅓ cup fresh dill, chopped
¼ cup fresh basil, roughly torn
Vinaigrette of choice
1 lime, quartered

Heat a grill or grill pan over medium-low heat. Rub zucchini, scallions, and chicken with oil; sprinkle with salt. Grill vegetables and chicken for about 20 minutes, until browned and cooked through, flipping once. Cut zucchini and scallions into a medium dice. Slice avocado in half, discard pit, and dice. Break chicken into large pieces. Toss grilled vegetables with lettuce, avocado, cilantro, and basil. Place on a large platter and drizzle with vinaigrette of choice; serve with lime quarters.

Makes 2 servings.

MAGGIE'S GARLIC LOVER'S KALE–GOAT CHEESE SPREAD

½ bunch kale
1 shallot
Extra virgin olive oil
1 clove garlic
1 to 2 oz soft goat cheese

Lightly sauté kale and shallot in olive oil. Transfer to food processor; toss in garlic and a splash more of olive oil. Blend well, then add goat cheese and blend again until mixed together. Enjoy this spread on French bread, rye crackers, or multigrain bread.

Makes 6 to 8 servings.

MARISE'S HEALTHY VEGGIE PANCAKES

3 egg whites
2 zucchini, grated
2 oz goat mozzarella, grated (blot with a paper towel to remove excess liquid)
1 tbsp minced onion
1 tbsp chia seeds
Freshly ground black pepper

Beat egg whites and mix in remaining ingredients very carefully so as to not overbeat the eggs or break the zucchini. Shape into 6 to 8 small pancakes and spoon into a nonstick frying pan. Cook for 3 to 4 minutes, then flip to other side and cook for another 3 to 4 minutes, until golden brown.

Makes 6 to 8 small pancakes, or 2 to 3 servings.

MOCK "SPINACH" DIP (VEGAN)

1 small zucchini
1 medium potato
1 small bunch kale
¼ tsp sea salt
1 to 2 tbsp onion flakes
½ tsp dried thyme
1 tsp dried parsley
2 cloves garlic, pressed
Freshly ground black pepper, to taste

Steam the zucchini and potato until tender and drain thoroughly (if you have thyroid dysfunction, you can steam the kale as well). Combine zucchini, potato, and ¾ of the kale, and puree in food processor; add seasonings, garlic, and black pepper, and blend. If the consistency is too thick, add more kale; if not, you can use leftover kale for salad. Chill overnight before serving.

Makes 10 to 12 servings.

SPICY BRUSCHETTA

Extra virgin olive oil
Chili flakes or lemon zest or orange zest
Parmesan, shaved
Garlic, chopped
Baguette slices (a large baguette will make approximately 30 slices; you can always freeze baguettes!)
Grilled or sautéed vegetables (grilled zucchini with fresh basil or sautéed shiitakes are great options)

Combine olive oil with chili flakes or lemon zest or orange zest, Parmesan, and chopped garlic. Toast baguette slices and brush liberally with spiced oil, then add vegetable toppings.

Makes 15 servings.

HOMEMADE GUACAMOLE

2 ripe avocados
½ red onion, minced (about ½ cup)
1 jalapeño pepper
Juice of ½ lime
⅛ tsp sea salt
Freshly ground black pepper
Optional: add roasted jalapeño and/or 2 tbsp cilantro, chopped

Cut avocados in half, remove pit, and scoop out and mash the avocado fruit. Add onion, jalapeño, lime juice, and salt and pepper, and mash some more. Finish by adding optional ingredients, if desired. For a creamier texture, add water. If not serving immediately, keep avocado pit in to prevent guacamole from turning brown and store in refrigerator in a covered container for up to 3 days.

Makes 8 to 10 servings.

SPICED COCONUT SPINACH AND POTATOES

1 shallot
1 large clove garlic
¼ tsp fine-grain sea salt
1 tbsp ghee, extra virgin olive oil, or grape-seed oil
¼ tsp whole cumin seeds
¼ tsp red pepper flakes
2 medium potatoes, thinly sliced
7 oz organic spinach, well washed, chopped
1 yellow squash, chopped
Squeeze of lemon
1½ tbsp unsweetened shredded coconut, lightly toasted

Place shallot and garlic on a cutting board; sprinkle with salt and chop or mash into a paste. Heat ghee or oil in your largest skillet over medium heat. Stir in cumin seeds and red pepper flakes and cook for 1 minute, then stir in shallot-garlic paste and potatoes. Sauté until potatoes soften, then add spinach and squash. Keep stirring until spinach starts collapsing a bit and brightens up (about 1 minute). Finish with lemon juice and coconut.

Makes 2 to 3 servings.

SPINACH SALAD WITH NUTS AND CHEESE (WARM)

3 tbsp raw walnuts
8 cups baby kale, washed
2 oz goat cheese or 1 oz Manchego
⅛ cup golden raisins, dried cranberries
2 tbsp red onion, minced
Dressing of choice

Heat nuts in a dry skillet, stirring occasionally, for 30 seconds, or until they are golden brown. Sauté spinach for about 1 minute, or until it is wilted. Add cheese, raisins or dried cranberries, and onion, and combine with dressing of choice.

Makes 2 to 3 servings.

SPRING ROLLS

3 large lettuce leaves, torn into strips
1 cucumber, sliced into thin strips
½ cup shredded zucchini
2 green onions, chopped
1 carrot, grated
1 cup cooked rice vermicelli or bean thread noodles
2 tbsp fresh cilantro
2 tbsp fresh basil
1 cup water, approximately
6 to 8 spring roll wrappers

Combine all ingredients except water, some cilantro and basil leaves, and spring roll wrappers in a large bowl and toss well. Place water in a shallow pan. Dip spring roll wrappers in water until pliable, 1 at a time. Fill each wrapper with 2 to 3 tbsp of vegetable filling. Place 2 or 3 basil and cilantro leaves on top and roll up.

Makes 6 to 8 servings.

HOMEMADE HUMMUS

2 cups drained well-cooked or canned low-sodium chickpeas, liquid reserved
¼ cup extra virgin olive oil, plus oil for drizzling
2 cloves garlic, peeled
Sea salt and freshly ground black pepper to taste
1 tbsp ground cumin, or to taste, plus a sprinkling for garnish
Juice of 1 lemon
Chopped fresh parsley leaves for garnish

Put all ingredients except parsley in a food processor and begin to process. Add chickpea liquid or water as needed to produce a smooth puree.

Taste and adjust the seasonings (you may want to add more lemon juice). Serve drizzled with olive oil and sprinkled with a bit more cumin and some parsley.

Makes 8 to 10 servings.

THAI CHICKEN SOUP

4 quarts water
4 whole chicken legs, cut into quarters
2 stalks celery, sliced into 2-inch pieces (can include leaves for extra
    flavor)
2 whole carrots, coarsely chopped
1 leek, chopped
1 onion, chopped
3 cloves garlic
1 bunch kale
¼ can coconut milk
2 tbsp grated fresh ginger
Cinnamon to taste
½ tsp sea salt
Freshly ground black pepper
Sriracha sauce to taste
Optional: lemongrass

Fill a large pot with 4 quarts water; place over high heat and bring
to a boil. Add chicken and return to a boil, skimming off any foam
that accumulates on top. Reduce heat to low and continue cooking,
uncovered, for 2 hours. Add remaining ingredients except for Sriracha
sauce and lemongrass, and continue cooking slowly, uncovered,
for 1 hour. Remove layer of fat that has formed on top of soup. Adjust
seasonings. If desired, add in lemongrass stalk and let simmer for an
additional 10 minutes.

Makes 6 to 8 servings.

WATERCRESS AND APPLE SALAD

3 medium-sized apples
1 tbsp lime juice, plus a squeeze more for apple
¼ cup plain yogurt
2 tbsp raw almond butter
1 tbsp water
⅛ tsp sea salt
Freshly ground black pepper to taste
2 to 3 bunches watercress (cut off and discard stems)

Dice apple and toss with squeeze of lime (this will help keep apple from browning). Whisk together yogurt, nut butter, water, 1 tbsp lime juice, salt, and pepper, and toss with watercress and apple.

Makes 4 servings.

WATERMELON, GOAT CHEESE, AND ARUGULA SALAD

2 cups diced watermelon
3 cups arugula
3 oz goat cheese (hard or soft), crumbled
Orange Oil (see page 176)
Freshly ground black pepper

Combine watermelon and arugula, then add goat cheese. Drizzle with Orange Oil and top with pepper.

Try this variation: watermelon and arugula with basil and mozzarella. Fresh, unsalted mozzarella is one of the cleanest cow's milk cheeses you can have!

Makes 2 to 3 servings.

WILD MUSHROOM CROSTINI

3 cups diced oyster mushrooms
3 cups diced shiitake mushrooms
2 to 3 tbsp extra virgin olive oil or truffle oil
Sea salt and freshly ground black pepper
Baguette slices (a large baguette will make approximately 30 slices; you
    can always freeze baguettes!)
Optional: grated goat Parmesan or Pecorino Romano

Sauté mushrooms in oil; season with salt and pepper. Slice baguette
and toast in oven, then spoon mushroom mixture on top. Optional:
top with grated Parmesan.

Makes 15 servings.

VEGAN CHICKEN STOCK (OR NOT)

1 onion
4 cloves garlic
2 tbsp extra virgin olive oil
1 tbsp poultry seasoning
¼ tsp sea salt
1 bay leaf
Freshly ground black pepper
Cinnamon to taste
Optional: fresh chopped ginger to taste
Optional: chili flakes to taste
1 to 2 tsp honey
4 quarts water
Optional: 1 whole chicken, cut up

Sauté onion and garlic until lightly browned; add all seasonings (including ginger and chili flakes, if desired) except honey. Stir for 2 minutes.
Add honey and then water. Add chicken, if desired. Let simmer for at
least 2 hours for a rich broth; skim off foam and fat. For vegetarian version, when serving soup, top each serving with 1 tbsp butter.

Makes 6 to 8 servings.

JENNIFER'S FLAXSEED TREATS

These are great with hot cereal or as a sweet snack.

1 cup flaxseeds (about 6 oz)
3 tbsp packed light brown sugar
3 tbsp honey
Optional: pinch of ground cinnamon and/or ground ginger

Soak flaxseeds overnight in ½ cup water. Spread in a thin layer on a baking sheet and bake at 275 °F, turning several times to dry out (50 minutes to 1 hour).

Spray liberally with cooking spray 2 large sheets of waxed or parchment paper. (You can also use a cookie sheet or baking pan.) In small saucepan, combine brown sugar and honey over low heat. Stir constantly until sugar is melted and mixture is thick. Cook for about 5 minutes for a chewy texture; cooking for about 7 minutes will give a harder texture to the treat. Stir in flaxseeds with wooden spoon until well coated. Scrape mixture onto 1 piece of greased paper. Top with second sheet, greased side down. Use a rolling pin to flatten mixture to about ¼ inch thick. Remove top sheet. Let treats cool, then break apart. Store in airtight container.

Makes 10 to 12 servings.

PUMPKIN–SUNFLOWER SEED SNACK MIX

1 cup raw pumpkin seeds
1 cup raw sunflower seeds
Sprinkling of Maine Coast Sea Seasoning
Freshly ground black pepper
1 tbsp garlic powder
2 tbsp extra virgin olive oil

Combine ingredients in plastic bag and shake until seeds are well coated. Roast at 175 °F for 15 to 20 minutes, or until lightly browned.

Makes 8 to 10 servings.

REGINA'S RAW CORN TORTILLA CHIPS

¼ cup whole flaxseeds
¾ to 1 cup water
1 bag frozen organic corn, thawed and drained
½ white onion
1 clove garlic
Cumin or other preferred seasoning, to taste

Place flaxseeds in a bowl and stir in water. Let soak until water is absorbed, 1 to 2 hours. Preheat oven to lowest setting (around 120 °F). In a blender, puree corn, onion, garlic, and seasoning. Combine corn puree with flaxseeds and spread evenly on a baking sheet or other shallow pan (it's best to use a Silpat or similar silicone liner). Bake until mixture is completely dehydrated and breaks crisply (this can take all day). For a thinner chip and less time, divide between 2 baking sheets.

Makes 6 servings.

KATIE'S KALE CHIPS

1 bunch kale, chopped
1 tbsp extra virgin olive oil
Pinch of sea salt
Freshly ground black pepper
Optional: 1 tbsp chili flakes
Fresh lime juice

Preheat oven to lowest setting (around 120 °F). Make sure Kale is dry, then coat lightly in olive oil and add salt, pepper, and chili flakes, if desired. Add lime juice at the end. Spread kale on a baking sheet and bake for 40 minutes to 1 hour.

Makes 4 to 8 servings.

SHIITAKE PATE

9 ounces shiitake mushrooms
¼ cup cup extra virgin olive oil or truffle oil (divided in half)
1 tbsp Italian herbs or Herbes de Provence
⅛ cup sunflower seeds or walnuts
Dash of sea salt

Slow sauté shiitakes in ⅛ cup of the oil and the tbsp of herbs until they create jus. Place in food processor with seeds or nuts, dash of salt, and remaining oil and puree until smooth. Serve with bruschetta or crackers.

Makes 10 to 12 servings.

SIDE DISHES

BLUE POTATOES

Blue or Peruvian potatoes are moderate in starch but *very* high in antioxidants and make great roasted potatoes. If you would like potatoes lower in starch, substitute fingerling potatoes.

4 blue potatoes
¼ cup extra virgin olive oil
Italian herbs, to taste
Sea salt
Freshly ground black pepper
3 cloves garlic, chopped
1 small onion, chopped

Preheat oven to 425 °F. Cut potatoes into cubes and toss with remaining ingredients. Spread on a baking sheet and roast for 30 minutes.

Makes 8 servings.

JOANNA'S BUTTERNUT SQUASH

1 large butternut squash
1 tsp smoked sweet paprika
1 tsp garlic powder
1 tsp onion powder
1 tsp freshly ground black pepper
3 tbsp extra virgin olive oil
2 tsp balsamic vinegar

Preheat oven to 375 °F. Cut ends off butternut squash, peel, and slice lengthwise. Remove seeds and chop into 1-inch cubes. In a medium bowl, combine seasonings, oil, and vinegar into a paste. Add squash and toss until coated. Arrange squash cubes in 1 layer in a roasting pan. Roast for 20 minutes, toss once, and roast for an additional 25 minutes, or until squash is browned and tender throughout.

Makes 4 servings.

VEGETABLE FRIES

4 medium carrots, cut into ½-inch-thick sticks
1 small rutabaga, peeled and cut into ½-inch-thick sticks
2 to 3 tbsp extra virgin olive oil
Sea salt
Freshly ground black pepper

Heat oven to 450 °F. Toss vegetables with olive oil, salt, and pepper, and roast on a baking sheet for 20 to 25 minutes, tossing once.

Makes 6 to 8 servings.

DINNER

AFRICAN APPLE-PEANUT STEW

1 to 2 bunches collard greens; if you have thyroid dysfunction, use kale
   (4 to 8 cups, sliced) and almonds
2 tbsp extra virgin olive oil
1 large onion, chopped
2 garlic cloves, minced or pressed
2 cups chopped apple
½ cup water
½ cup peanut butter
1 tbsp Tabasco or other hot pepper sauce
¼ cup chopped parsley
Sea salt to taste
Crushed skinless peanuts
Chopped scallions
Cooked rice or other grain as an accompaniment

Prepare kale and almonds or collard greens by washing it and removing large center stem from each leaf. Stack leaves on a cutting board and slice into 1-inch slices.

In a large wok with a cover, or a Dutch oven (nonstick preferred), heat olive oil and sauté onion for about 6 minutes, stirring frequently, until lightly browned. Add garlic and stir for 1 minute.

Add apples and water to onions and bring to a simmer. Stir in collard greens or kale, cover, and simmer for about 5 minutes, stirring a couple of times, until just tender. Mix in peanut butter, Tabasco, and parsley, and simmer for 5 minutes. Add salt to taste, and serve topped with crushed peanuts and scallions, over rice or other grain.

Makes 4 servings.

AMY'S VEGGIE SANDWICH

¼ avocado
Whole grain bread
¼ shredded carrot
Cucumber slices
Sunflower seeds
Mixed greens

Spread avocado on 1 slice of bread, then layer on carrot, cucumber, sunflower, seeds, and greens.

Makes 1 serving.

ARCTIC CHAR WITH TARRAGON AND ORANGE OIL

3 long sprigs fresh tarragon
⅓ tsp sea salt
4 tbsp Orange Oil (page 176)
1 lb Arctic char
Juice of 1 orange

Mix together tarragon sprigs, salt, and oil. Massage mixture gently into fish and let marinate for at least 2 hours. Squeeze orange juice onto fish and broil on high for 6 to 8 minutes, depending on thickness of fish.

Makes 2 to 4 servings.

BAKED "FRIED" CHICKEN

Seasonings of choice (jerk seasoning, barbecue seasoning, smoked chipotles with cinnamon, Herbes de Provence, etc.)
2 cups panko
1 lb chicken thighs, with or without skin

Add seasoning of choice to panko. Coat chicken with seasoned panko (no need to use egg). Bake at 400 °F for 30 minutes in cast-iron skillet. Turn once and bake for an additional 10 minutes.

Makes 4 servings.

BOURBON DUCK BREASTS WITH APPLES

Juice of 1 lemon

2 firm apples, such as Fuji

1½ lb duck breast (or approximately 2 breasts; portion size per serving is 4 to 6 ounces for women and 6 to 8 for men)

3 tbsp duck fat

1 tbsp brown sugar

½ cup bourbon

2 tbsp finely chopped orange zest

Sea salt

Squeeze lemon juice into a bowl. Slice apples into quarter moons, about ⅛ inch thick. Do not peel. Drop each slice into lemon juice and make sure all sides are coated to avoid browning.

Score the duck breasts by cutting an "X" into the skin. Heat a large sauté pan over high heat for 1 to 2 minutes. Add duck breasts, skin side down; lower heat to medium and cook for 5 to 8 minutes, until golden brown. Turn over and cook for another 2 to 4 minutes, depending on how you like your duck. Remove duck breasts and place on a plate to collect the drippings. Let them rest for 5 to 10 minutes. Pour off all but 3 tablespoons of fat from the pan.

Cook apples over medium heat in remaining duck fat (do not crowd apples). Brown them lightly on both sides. When you have flipped them, sprinkle brown sugar over pan and swirl to combine while apples continue to cook for 1 to 2 minutes. Remove apples and place on a paper towel.

Pour bourbon, leftover duck jus, and orange zest into pan and turn heat to high. Sprinkle a pinch of sea salt in pan and boil until mixture has cooked down by two-thirds.

Slice duck breast pieces roughly the same width as apples. To serve, make a rosette of alternating slices of duck breast and apple in center of each plate. Spoon a small amount of reduced sauce over each piece of duck.

Makes 4 servings.

SPICY ORANGE BEEF STIR-FRY

Zest and juice of 1 orange
¼ tsp coarse sea salt
1 tbsp Chinese rice wine
1 tsp honey or agave nectar
1 lb beef, chopped for stir-fry
2 tbsp extra virgin olive oil
3 to 4 cloves garlic, sliced
2 inches of fresh ginger, peeled and grated
Chili flakes, to taste
⅓ cup water
3 to 4 cups of broccoli florets
½ cup sliced scallion greens

Zest orange and set aside. Squeeze juice from orange into a bowl. Add salt, rice wine, and honey or agave nectar, and stir to combine; set aside.

Stir-fry beef for 1 minute in 1 tbsp of the olive oil. Transfer to a plate and set aside.

Add remaining olive oil to pan; add garlic, ginger, and chili flakes, and stir-fry for about 30 seconds. Add water, bell pepper, and broccoli. Cook for 4 to 5 minutes, then add orange zest mix. Add beef and scallions and sauté for 1 additional minute, or to desired doneness.

Makes 4 servings.

CHICKEN MOLE

2 tbsp olive oil
1 onion, chopped
3 cloves garlic, chopped
2 tbsp chili powder
1 tsp ground cumin
1 tsp ground cinnamon
Freshly ground black pepper
2 chipotle peppers, roughly chopped
4 oz red wine
4 oz low-sodium chicken stock or vegan broth
2 ounces bittersweet chocolate, chopped
1 whole chicken, cut into 8 pieces

Preheat oven to 400 °F.

For sauce:

Heat oil in a sauté pan over medium heat. Add onion and sauté until translucent. Add garlic and spices and continue to sauté 1 to 2 minutes more, to toast and develop flavor. Add chipotles, wine, stock, and chocolate. Simmer for 10 minutes. Strain and puree until smooth.

For chicken:

Sear chicken in a heavy-bottomed hot sauté pan over medium-high heat until browned on both sides. Put in a baking dish or casserole, cover with sauce, and braise in preheated oven for 45 minutes.

Makes 8 servings.

PANKO FRIED FISH (OR CHICKEN)

1 lb fish or chicken
1 cup panko bread crumbs
Seasonings of choice (jerk seasoning, Italian herb blend, Indian Spice Rub, etc.)
2 tbsp extra virgin olive oil
Optional: lemon, parsley, or cilantro

Cut fish or chicken into strips. Combine panko with 3 to 4 tbsp of seasoning of choice. Dredge fish or chicken in seasoned panko. Heat olive oil in a large skillet over medium heat; sauté fish or chicken. Garnish with lemon, parsley, or cilantro, as desired.

Makes 4 servings.

JILL'S SIMPLE LAMB CURRY

2 lb lean lamb shoulder, cut into ¾-inch cubes
1 tbsp grated fresh ginger
1½ tsp grated garlic
1½ tsp turmeric
½ tsp cumin seeds, toasted and ground
½ tsp coriander seeds, toasted and ground
¼ tsp cayenne
Sea salt
2 tbsp ghee or grape-seed oil
2 red onions, sliced thick
½ tsp cloves
10 black peppercorns
1-inch piece cinnamon stick
2 cups water

Put lamb in a bowl with ginger, garlic, turmeric, cumin, coriander, cayenne, and salt; mix well. Marinate at room temperature 30 minutes, or up to several hours refrigerated (even overnight is fine).

Heat ghee or oil in a heavy-bottomed soup pot or Dutch oven over medium heat. Add onions and cook for 3 to 4 minutes, until softened. Raise heat to medium-high and add seasoned lamb. Lightly brown lamb and onions, stirring occasionally, for another 5 minutes or so. Add cloves, peppercorns, and cinnamon stick, then add water and bring to a boil. Cover pot and turn heat to low. Simmer gently for about 1 hour, or until meat is fork-tender. Add salt to taste. Raise heat and reduce sauce a bit, if desired. (May be prepared ahead to this point and reheated before serving.)

Makes 6 to 8 servings.

LAMB SHEPHERD'S PIE

1 lb ground lamb
1 tbsp extra virgin olive oil
1 onion, chopped
3 cloves garlic, chopped
1 zucchini, chopped
½ bunch kale, chopped into 1-inch strips
1 medium potato, chopped into 1-inch cubes
1 medium butternut squash, chopped into 1-inch cubes
4 oz butter
½ cup full-fat coconut milk
Cinnamon, cayenne, cumin, and turmeric, or herbs of choice
Coarse sea salt

Sauté lamb in oil with onion and garlic until browned. Add zucchini and simmer for 10 minutes. Add kale and cover; turn off heat and let steam for 5 to 8 minutes.

In a separate pot, steam potato and squash. Separate potatoes and squash into 2 bowls. Add 2 oz of butter and ¼ cup of coconut milk to each and mash until creamy. Add seasonings of choice and salt to taste.

Layer a casserole dish with potato mixture, lamb/kale mixture, and butternut squash mixture. Bake at 400 °F for 15 minutes.

Makes 6 servings.

LINDSEY'S VEGGIE BURGER

½ cup basmati rice (doubled if you like more rice)
½ cup lentils
1 tsp plus 1 tbsp extra virgin olive oil, plus more for cooking burgers
1 onion, diced small
½ cup shiitake mushrooms, diced small
3 large red beets (about 1 lb), diced small
3 to 4 cloves garlic, minced
1 tbsp lemon juice
1 chipotle, chopped
2 tbsp golden flaxseeds
1 tbsp pumpkin seeds
Optional: sliced cheese

Cook rice and lentils so they are a bit mushy (overcooked). Heat 1 tsp olive oil in a skillet over medium-high heat. Add onion, reduce heat to medium, and cook until onions are translucent and softened. Add mushrooms and cook until tender (another 10 minutes or so). Stir in beets. Cover and cook until beets are completely tender, stirring occasionally. Add garlic and cook until it is fragrant, about 30 seconds. Deglaze pan using lemon juice. Add 1 tbsp olive oil and chipotle. Stir to combine, then adjust seasonings. Add flaxseeds and pumpkin seeds as a glue and stir a bit more to combine and cook seeds. Add vegetables to rice and lentils and mix.

Heat a cast-iron skillet over highest heat. Add a few teaspoons of olive oil; oil should completely coat bottom of pan. When you see oil shimmer and it flows easily, pan is ready.

Using your hands, scoop up about 1 cup of burger mixture and shape it into a patty. Set patty in pan, where it should begin to sizzle immediately (if it doesn't sizzle, wait 1 or 2 minutes before cooking the rest of the burgers). Shape and add as many more patties as will fit loosely in your pan. Once all patties are in pan, reduce heat to medium-high.

Cook patties for 2 minutes, then flip them. You should see a nice crust on cooked side. If they break apart a little when flipped, just reshape them with spatula; they'll hold together once second side is cooked. If you're adding cheese, lay a slice over each burger now. Cook second side for another 2 minutes.

Cooked burgers should be eaten the same day. You can also save leftover uncooked mixture in refrigerator for up to 1 week in a closed container and cook just 1 or 2 burgers as you want them.

Makes 8 to 10 burgers.

MAGGIE'S MOM'S SOLE ALMONDINE

For fish:

2 cups all-purpose flour
Pinch of sea salt
Freshly ground black pepper
1 cup Silk coconut milk or Rice Dream
2 sole fillets
1 egg
2 tbsp unsalted butter
1 tbsp extra virgin olive oil

For sauce:

1 tbsp butter
1 tbsp extra virgin olive oil
2 cups blanched slivered almonds

For garnish:

1 lemon, cut into wedges
Chopped flat-leaf parsley

Season flour with salt and pepper. Fill a shallow plate or bowl with milk and place fillets in bowl for 2 minutes. Beat egg with a little water. Transfer fillets to egg mixture.

Lightly dredge fillets in flour mixture. Place fillets, covered with wax paper, in refrigerator for 10 to 15 minutes to allow flour mixture to adhere.

Heat butter and olive oil in a pan. When it's hot, sauté sole, turning once, 2 minutes on each side over medium heat (depending on thickness of fillets). Place on paper towel on a plate.

For sauce, add butter and olive oil to pan and sauté almonds until golden brown. To serve, sprinkle almonds over fillets and garnish with lemon wedge and parsley.

Makes 4 servings.

PAN-SEARED FIVE-SPICE DUCK BREAST
WITH BALSAMIC JUS

1 large garlic clove, finely chopped
1 tbsp grated fresh ginger
2 tsp five-spice powder
1 tsp sea salt
½ tsp freshly ground black pepper
4 single duck breasts
1 tbsp extra virgin olive oil
¼ cup dry red wine
2 tbsp balsamic vinegar

In a large, heavy, self-sealing plastic bag, combine garlic, ginger, five-spice powder, salt, and pepper. Add duck breasts, seal, shake to coat duck breast, and refrigerate for at least 1 hour and up to 24 hours. Remove from refrigerator 1 hour before cooking.

Preheat oven to 400 °F. In a large ovenproof sauté pan, heat olive oil over medium-high heat until shimmering. Score the duck breast and sear skin side down, for 5 minutes; turn and sear for 5 minutes on other side. Transfer pan to oven and roast for 5 minutes for medium-rare. Transfer duck breasts to a plate and keep warm.

To make balsamic jus, pour off fat from pan. Return pan to medium-high heat, add wine, and stir to scrape up browned bits from bottom of pan. Cook to reduce wine by half. Add balsamic vinegar and cook to reduce for several more minutes.

Cut duck breasts into diagonal slices and serve drizzled with balsamic jus.

Makes 6 to 8 servings.

SARAH'S LOW-REACTIVE PASTA

1¼ cups all-purpose white flour (not using pasta flour decreases chance of reactivity)
2 eggs, lightly beaten
Sea salt

Sift flour, mound it on work surface with a well in center, and pour eggs into well. Use your fingers to incorporate eggs into flour and knead for 10 minutes. Shape dough into a ball and let sit 15 minutes.

Roll out on lightly floured surface to make a thin sheet and cut into desired shapes or pass through a pasta machine. It's a good idea to let pasta shapes dry for 20 minutes or so, then boil in lightly salted water for 4 to 5 minutes. Serve with your choice of sauce.

Makes 4 servings.

TEMPEH BURGERS

1 package tempeh
1 tart apple (such as Granny Smith or Fuji)
1 egg
Maine Coast Sea Seasonings Salt (Dulse w/Garlic flavor)
1 tsp sage (dry or fresh)
¼ red onion
¼ cup panko
Extra virgin olive oil
Splash of water if needed

Grate tempeh in a food processor. Shred apple in food processor. Combine tempeh and apple with all remaining ingredients in a bowl and mix well. Shape into burgers and pan-fry them in olive oil over low heat for 4 to 5 minutes per side, or until golden brown.

Makes 6 to 8 servings.

VANESSA'S ZUCCHINI "PIZZA"

1 large zucchini
Extra virgin olive oil
2 to 3 cloves garlic, chopped
2 tsp fresh rosemary, chopped
2 tbsp chopped fresh basil leaves
6 oz fresh, unsalted mozzarella, shredded

Slice zucchini lengthwise, place on a broiler or grill pan, and brush with olive oil. Broil or grill zucchini until browned and tender but not too soggy; remove from pan. Add garlic to rosemary and coat zucchini lightly. Return zucchini to pan, sprinkle basil leaves over, cover with mozzarella, and place back under broiler or on grill until cheese is melted.

Makes 6 servings.

DESSERTS

CARROT CAKE

2 cups firmly packed finely grated carrots
Juice of 1 large orange
2 tsp vanilla extract
¼ cup light olive oil
1 cup honey, liquefied in microwave for 30 seconds
2½ cups unbleached all-purpose white flour
2 tsp baking soda
1 tsp cinnamon
½ tsp allspice
Optional: ¾ cup raw walnuts, chopped

Preheat oven to 350 °F. In a mixing bowl, stir together carrots, orange juice, vanilla, olive oil, and honey until well blended.

In another bowl, stir together flour, baking soda, and spices. Mix in walnuts, if desired. Blend dry ingredients into carrot mixture, stirring until just combined.

Pour batter into a nonstick 8-inch-square baking pan and bake for 45 minutes to 1 hour, until a knife inserted in center comes out clean. Remove from oven, let cool slightly, and remove from pan. Slice into 8 to 12 pieces.

Makes 8 to 12 servings.

CHOCOLATE-COVERED STRAWBERRIES

5 oz bittersweet chocolate, chopped
1 pint fresh strawberries with hulls

In a microwave-safe bowl, heat chocolate until melted (time will vary according to strength of microwave). Stir occasionally until chocolate is smooth. Holding berries by hulls, dip each in molten chocolate, about ¾ of the way to the hull. Place, hull side down, on wax paper and chill until set.

2 strawberries equals 1 serving.

CREAMY CHOCOLATE-COFFEE POPS

¼ cup agave nectar or honey
⅛ cup water
1 tsp cocoa powder
1 cup strong French roast coffee
2 tbsp heavy cream

Combine all ingredients in a blender. Put mixture into four ice pop molds, insert sticks, and freeze for 5 hours or longer.

Makes 4 servings.

FLOURLESS ALMOND COOKIES

2 cups whole blanched almonds (plus 24 additional blanched almonds)
⅛ cup sugar
1 tsp vanilla extract
Dash of sea salt
1 large egg
4 tbsp chia seeds
1 tsp cinnamon

Preheat oven to 350 °F. Place 2 cups almonds in food processor and grind fine. Add sugar, vanilla, salt, and egg, and chia seeds, and pulse until dough forms into a ball.

Divide dough into 24 balls, about 1 tbsp each. Place on baking sheets prepared with cooking spray and sprinkle with cinnamon. Gently press 1 whole almond into center of each cookie. Bake for 15 minutes and let cool on sheet for 5 minutes.

Makes 24 cookies.

HOMEMADE NUTELLA

1 cup hazelnuts
¼ cup cocoa powder
5 tbsp agave nectar
1 tbsp vanilla extract
1 tbsp hazelnut oil
Pinch of sea salt

Preheat oven to 350 °F. Roast hazelnuts on a baking sheet for 8 to 10 minutes, until they darken a bit and smell fragrant. Transfer to a towel and rub off skins as much as you can. In a food processor, grind hazelnuts for about 5 minutes to a smooth butter. Add cocoa, agave nectar, vanilla, oil, and salt and process about 1 minute, or until well blended. Stores best in a glass Mason jar in refrigerator, up to 1 week.

FROZEN RICOTTA COOKIE SANDWICHES

1 cup fresh ricotta

2 tsp honey

Optional seasonings: ½ tsp lavender, vanilla extract, orange zest, or lemon zest

Optional toppings: hazelnuts, almond slivers, coconut or chocolate shavings, Homemade Nutella (see preceding recipe)

16 graham crackers

In a food processor, combine ricotta and honey with flavoring of choice. Using an ice cream scoop, divide into 8 portions and place on wax paper. Freeze for several hours. To make sandwiches, place one scoop of ice cream on graham cracker, add tested topping if desired, top with another graham cracker, and serve.

Makes 8 servings.

RAW VEGAN CHOCOLATE MACAROONS

1 cup grated unsweetened coconut

½ overripe banana, mashed

⅛ cup coconut oil

1 tbsp agave nectar or honey

2 tbsp cocoa powder

Optional: orange zest or Orange Oil (page 176)

Mix all ingredients and form into 8 mounds; no need to bake.

Makes 8 macaroons.

REBECCA'S ALMOND JOY BARK

10-oz bag of dark chocolate chips

2 tbsp coconut oil

½ cup shredded unsweetened coconut

¼ cup chopped or sliced almonds

In a microwave or double boiler, melt chocolate chips with coconut oil. Stir mixture until smooth and pour into a baking pan lined with parchment or waxed paper. Sprinkle with coconut and almonds. Refrigerate until set, about 30 minutes. Cut into squares.

Makes 8 to 10 servings.

WATERMELON LIME POPS

2 cups watermelon
2 tbsp lime juice
2 tbsp honey

Combine ingredients in a blender and pour into four ice pop molds. Insert sticks and freeze for 5 hours or longer.

Makes 4 servings.

Part Five

ADDITIONAL PLAN MATERIALS

Spring Menu

The Spring Menu is what we use when the weather gets warm (or for those of us who live in a consistently warm climate), as the body responds differently to hot and cold foods with changing temperatures. As with the Winter Menu, the first three days of the Spring Menu consist of a detox cleanse, which resets your body by decreasing inflammation and creating a purified, neutral base line against which you'll begin testing new foods. Days Four through Twenty are the testing phase, when we begin to systematically test foods, starting with the least reactive.

I encourage you to read through Part Two for more insight into each phase, as well as answers to commonly asked questions, cooking tips, and more. For detailed information on each new food we test, please refer to the corresponding day in the regular menu listed in Part Two.

Note: You can download new days 1–20 at www.lyngenet.com.

Day One: No Test

UPON AWAKENING

- Weigh yourself and record the results in your Plan Journal.
- Drink 16 ounces of fresh water with lemon juice (after you weigh yourself).

- Take your liver support supplement and/or drink a cup of dandelion tea.

BREAKFAST

For women: 1 cup of flax granola with ½ cup of blueberries
For men: 1½ cups of flax granola with 1 cup of blueberries
Silk coconut milk or Rice Dream

LUNCH

Carrot Ginger Soup (page 178) with chia seeds or sunflower seeds
Sautéed or steamed broccoli drizzled with Orange Oil (page 176)
    and lemon juice (make enough to have some left over for
    lunch on Day Two)
Mixed greens with ½ pear and pumpkin seeds

SNACK

1 apple

DINNER

Sautéed Kale with Vegetables (page 178; make enough to have
    some left over for dinner on Day Two) with Spicy Coco Sauce
    (page 177)
Beet and Carrot Salad (page 178) with pumpkin seeds

WATER

Be sure to drink your recommended daily water intake throughout the day, ending by dinner.

Day Two: Almonds

UPON AWAKENING

- Weigh yourself and record the results in your Plan Journal.
- Drink 16 ounces of fresh water with lemon juice (after you weigh yourself).

- Take your liver support supplement and/or drink a cup of dandelion tea.

BREAKFAST

For women: 1 cup of flax granola with ½ cup of blueberries
For men: 1½ cups of flax granola with 1 cup of blueberries

LUNCH

Carrot Ginger Soup (page 178) with chia seeds or sunflower seeds
Mixed greens with ½ diced apple, ¼ avocado
Leftover sautéed or steamed broccoli with Orange Oil

SNACK

1 pear with a small handful of almonds

DINNER

Leftover Sautéed Kale with Vegetables with brown or basmati rice (1 cup for women, 1½ cups for men) with pumpkin seeds
Beet and Carrot Salad (page 178) with sunflower seeds (make enough to have some left over for dinner on Day Three)

WATER

Be sure to drink your recommended daily water intake throughout the day, ending by dinner.

Day Three: Chicken

UPON AWAKENING

- Weigh yourself and record the results in your Plan Journal.
- Drink 16 ounces of fresh water with lemon juice (after you weigh yourself).
- Take your liver support supplement and/or drink a cup of dandelion tea.

BREAKFAST

For women: 1 cup of flax granola with choice of ½ cup of blueberries or diced ½ pear

For men: 1½ cups of flax granola with choice of 1 cup of blueberries or 1 diced whole pear

LUNCH

Mixed greens with sunflowers seeds, ¼ avocado, and carrots

Cream of Broccoli Soup (page 294)

SNACK

1 to 2 cups of watermelon (optional: sprinkle with chia seeds)

DINNER

Chicken with Italian Herbs and Orange Zest (page 182; 2 to 3 ounces
for women, 4 ounces for men) on a bed of mixed greens

Steamed or sautéed zucchini, broccoli, carrots, onions, garlic, and
Italian herbs; finish with Orange Oil (page 176) and freshly
ground black pepper (make enough to have some left over for
lunch on Day Four)

Leftover Beet and Carrot Salad

WATER

Be sure to drink your recommended daily water intake throughout the day, ending by 7:30 p.m.

Day Four: Cheese

*Note: Please be sure to read "The Inside Scoop on Day Four" on page
99 so you don't miss out on all the fun stuff that Day Four reintroduces in addition to cheese, like coffee and wine!*

UPON AWAKENING

- Weigh yourself and record the results in your Plan Journal.
- Drink 16 ounces of fresh water with lemon juice (after you weigh yourself).
- Take your liver support supplement and/or drink a cup of dandelion tea.

BREAKFAST

For women: 1 cup of flax granola with choice of ½ cup of blueberries or diced ½ pear

For men: 1½ cups of flax granola with choice of 1 cup of blueberries or 1 diced whole pear

LUNCH

Leftover steamed or sautéed vegetables on a bed of spinach with pumpkin seeds and goat cheese (hard or soft)

Note: You can microwave the leftover vegetables to wilt the raw spinach beneath and make the iron in the spinach more bioavailable.

SNACK

Carrots with up to 6 tablespoons of Homemade Guacamole (page 204) or raw almond butter (1 to 2 tablespoons for women, 3 to 4 tablespoons for men)

DINNER

Chicken with Mango Salsa (page 176)

Mixed greens with carrots

Steamed or sautéed broccoli with Orange Oil (page 176) and chili flakes

DESSERT

1 ounce of dark chocolate (65 percent cacao maximum) or Cinnamon Poached Fruit (page 185) with optional Katie's Whipped Coconut Cream (page 296)

WATER

Be sure to drink your recommended daily water intake through-out the day, ending by dinner.

Note: This is a good time to retest for yeast. Check your tongue tomorrow morning to see if it has a white coating, which indicates a yeast overgrowth—especially if you include balsamic vinegar and wine in your menu today.

Day Five: Rye

UPON AWAKENING

- Weigh yourself and record the results in your Plan Journal.
- Drink 16 ounces of fresh water with lemon juice (after you weigh yourself).
- Take your liver support supplement and/or drink a cup of dandelion tea.

BREAKFAST

For women: 1 cup of flax granola with choice of approved fruit (½ cup of blueberries, ½ apple, or ½ pear)

For men: 1½ cups of flax granola with choice of approved fruit (1 cup of blueberries or 1 whole apple or pear)

LUNCH

Mixed greens with carrots, ¼ avocado, pumpkin seeds, and goat cheese

For women: 1 rye cracker with 1 to 2 tablespoons of raw almond butter or Homemade Hummus (page 181)

For men: 3 rye crackers with 3 to 4 tablespoons of raw almond butter or Homemade Hummus (page 181)

SNACK

1 to 2 cups of watermelon

DINNER

Chicken with Spicy Apricot Glaze (page 177) on a bed of arugula
Sautéed, roasted, or grilled zucchini with onion and basil topped
with Orange Oil (page 176) and sheep's milk Parmesan

DESSERT

1 ounce of dark chocolate or Cinnamon Poached Fruit (page 185)
with optional Katie's Whipped Coconut Cream (page 296)

WATER

Be sure to drink your recommended daily water intake throughout the day, ending by dinner.

Day Six: Protein

UPON AWAKENING

- Weigh yourself and record the results in your Plan Journal.
- Drink 16 ounces of fresh water with lemon juice (after you
  weigh yourself).
- Take your liver support supplement and/or drink a cup of dandelion tea.

BREAKFAST

For women: 1 cup of flax granola with choice of approved fruit
For men: 1½ cups of flax granola with choice of approved fruit

LUNCH

Mixed greens with avocado, carrots, beets, and pumpkin seeds
For women: 1 rye cracker with 1 to 2 tablespoons of raw almond
butter
For men: 3 rye crackers with 3 to 4 tablespoons of raw almond
butter

SNACK

The Plan Trail Mix (page 293; ¼ cup for women, ½ cup for men)

DINNER

Choose one protein from the list below to test on a bed of mixed greens:

Grilled *wild* white fish
Steak
Lamb
Venison
Duck
Egg

Roasted Squash, Kale and Manchego Salad (page 179; make enough to have some left over for lunch on Day Seven)
Note: Please turn to page 105 to read more about the different animal protein sources and for cooking suggestions.

DESSERT

1 ounce of dark chocolate or Cinnamon Poached Fruit (page 185) with optional Katie's Whipped Coconut Cream (page 296)

WATER

Be sure to drink your recommended daily water intake throughout the day, ending by dinner.

Day Seven: Optional Test Hummus/Chickpeas

UPON AWAKENING

- Weigh yourself and record the results in your Plan Journal.
- Drink 16 ounces of fresh water with lemon juice (after you weigh yourself).

- Take your liver support supplement and/or drink a cup of dandelion tea.

BREAKFAST

For women: 1 cup of flax granola with choice of approved fruit
For men: 1½ cups of flax granola with choice of approved fruit

LUNCH

Leftover Roasted Squash, Kale, and Manchego Salad
Rye cracker with raw almond butter (1 cracker for women, 3 crackers for men)

SNACK

1 ounce of salt-free potato chips
Note: Check out why salt-free potato chips are encouraged on The Plan on page 111.
OR
Carrots with Homemade Hummus (page 181; 4 tablespoons for women, 6 to 7 tablespoons for men)

DINNER

Chicken with Lemon Garlic Sauce (page 175) on a bed of arugula
Sautéed, grilled, or steamed vegetables (broccoli, carrots, zucchini, onions, and shiitakes) with garlic and herbs of choice (make enough to have some left over for dinner on Day Eight)

DESSERT

1 ounce of dark chocolate or Cinnamon Poached Fruit (page 185) with optional Katie's Whipped Coconut Cream (page 296)

WATER

Be sure to drink your recommended daily water intake throughout the day, ending by dinner.

Day Eight: Bread

UPON AWAKENING

- Weigh yourself and record the results in your Plan Journal.
- Drink 16 ounces of fresh water with lemon juice (after you weigh yourself).
- Take your liver support supplement and/or drink a cup of dandelion tea.

BREAKFAST

For women: 1 cup of Blueberry Compote (page 291)
For men: 1½ to 2 cups of Blueberry Compote (page 291)

LUNCH

1 slice of whole wheat or white bread with cheese, sunflower seeds, and avocado
Note: Please do not use a multigrain bread; stick to plain white or wheat for this test. See page 116 for more information about bread.
Spinach salad with ½ diced apple

SNACK

Carrots with up to 6 tablespoons of Homemade Hummus if testing chickpeas (page 181) or raw almond butter (1 to 2 tablespoons for women, 3 to 4 tablespoons for men)

DINNER

Protein that has been tested on a bed of mixed greens
Leftover vegetables from Day Seven's dinner

DESSERT

1 ounce of dark chocolate or Cinnamon Poached Fruit (page 185) with optional Katie's Whipped Coconut Cream (page 296)

WATER

Be sure to drink your recommended daily water intake through-out the day, ending by dinner.

Day Nine: No Test

UPON AWAKENING

- Weigh yourself and record the results in your Plan Journal.
- Drink 16 ounces of fresh water with lemon juice (after you weigh yourself).
- Take your liver support supplement and/or drink a cup of dandelion tea.

BREAKFAST

For women: 1 cup of flax granola with choice of approved fruit

For men: 1½ cups of flax granola with choice of approved fruit

OR

For women: ¾ cup of cereal mixed with ¼ cup of flax granola and approved fruit

For men: 1½ cups of cereal mixed with ½ cup of flax granola and approved fruit

Note: Please avoid puffed rice cereals, as they impair digestion. For more information on rice cereal choices, see page 120.

OR

For women: 1 slice of bread with 2 tablespoons of raw almond butter and ½ piece of fruit (if you passed the bread test)

For men: 1 slice of bread with 3 to 4 tablespoons of raw almond butter and 1 whole piece of fruit

LUNCH

Sautéed kale with goat cheese, ¼ avocado, carrots, and sunflower seeds

Carrots with up to 4 tablespoons of raw almond butter

SNACK

1 Chocolate-Covered Pear Slice (page 182) with a small handful
of sunflower seeds

OR

Salt-free potato chips (1 ounce for women, 1½ ounces for men)

DINNER

Any approved protein (make sure to rotate)

The Plan Chopped Salad (page 181) (make enough to have some
left over for lunch on Day Ten)

Steamed broccoli with Lemon Oil (page 176) and freshly ground
black pepper

DESSERT

1 ounce of dark chocolate or Cinnamon Poached Fruit (page 185)
with optional Katie's Whipped Coconut Cream (page 296)

WATER

Be sure to drink your recommended daily water intake throughout the day, ending by dinner.

Day Ten: Test New Protein

UPON AWAKENING

- Weigh yourself and record the results in your Plan Journal.
- Drink 16 ounces of fresh water with lemon juice (after you
  weigh yourself).
- Take your liver support supplement and/or drink a cup of dandelion tea.

BREAKFAST

For women: Smoothic (page 174) and 1 rye cracker with almond
butter

For men: Smoothie (page 174) and 3 rye crackers with almond butter

OR

Blueberry Compote (page 291; 1 cup for women, 1½ to 2 cups
for men)

LUNCH

Leftover The Plan Chopped Salad with pumpkin seeds

SNACK

Rye cracker with goat cheese and apple slices (1 cracker for
women, 3 crackers for men)

DINNER

Test a new protein from the list below on a bed on a bed of arugula:

Grilled *wild* white fish

Steak

Lamb

Venison

Duck

Scallops

Pork

Cow's cheese

Lentils

Tempeh

Pinto beans

Egg

Sautéed kale or spinach with sunflower seeds, avocado, Lemon
Oil (page 176), and Manchego cheese (make enough to have
some left over for lunch on Day Eleven)

DESSERT

1 ounce of dark chocolate or Cinnamon Poached Fruit (page 185) with optional Katie's Whipped Coconut Cream (page 296)

WATER

Be sure to drink your recommended daily water intake throughout the day, ending by dinner.

Day Eleven: No Test

UPON AWAKENING

- Weigh yourself and record the results in your Plan Journal.
- Drink 16 ounces of fresh water with lemon juice (after you weigh yourself).
- Take your liver support supplement and/or drink a cup of dandelion tea.

BREAKFAST

For women: 1 cup of flax granola with choice of approved fruit
For men: 1½ cups of flax granola with choice of approved fruit
OR
Bread with raw almond butter and approved fruit

LUNCH

Leftover sautéed kale or spinach with apple, sunflower seeds, and optional soup of choice

SNACK

Salt-free potato chips (1 ounce for women, 1½ ounces for men)

DINNER

Any approved protein (make sure to rotate)

Vegetable Timbale (page 183; 1 cup for women, 2 cups for men; make enough to have some left over for lunch on Day Twelve)

Baby romaine lettuce with grated carrots and cucumbers (make enough to have some left over for dinner on Day Twelve)

DESSERT

1 ounce of dark chocolate or Cinnamon Poached Fruit (page 185) with optional Katie's Whipped Coconut Cream (page 296)

WATER

Be sure to drink your recommended daily water intake throughout the day, ending by dinner.

Day Twelve: Test New Vegetable

UPON AWAKENING

- Weigh yourself and record the results in your Plan Journal.
- Drink 16 ounces of fresh water with lemon juice (after you weigh yourself).
- Take your liver support supplement and/or drink a cup of dandelion tea.

BREAKFAST

Smoothie (page 174)

OR

Blueberry Compote (page 291; 1 cup for women, 1½ to 2 cups for men)

LUNCH

Leftover Vegetable Timbale (1 cup for women, 2 cups for men) and salad with pumpkin seeds

Rye cracker with raw almond butter (1 cracker for women, 3 crackers for men)

SNACK

For women: ½ piece of fruit with a small handful of almonds
For men: 1 whole piece of fruit with a small handful of almonds
OR
1 to 2 cups of watermelon (optional to add chia seeds)

DINNER

Approved protein (make sure to rotate)
Test a new vegetable mixed with other approved vegetables (sautéed, steamed, grilled, or roasted) and herbs of choice (make enough to have some left over for lunch on Day Thirteen)
Note: We always test a new vegetable mixed in with other approved vegetables to minimize the chance of reactivity. For more on this and a list of lower-reactive vegetable choices, please see page 129.
Leftover baby romaine salad

DESSERT

1 ounce of dark chocolate or Cinnamon Poached Fruit (page 185) with optional Katie's Whipped Coconut Cream (page 296)

WATER

Be sure to drink your recommended daily water intake throughout the day, ending by dinner.

Day Thirteen: No Test

UPON AWAKENING

- Weigh yourself and record the results in your Plan Journal.
- Drink 16 ounces of fresh water with lemon juice (after you weigh yourself).
- Take your liver support supplement and/or drink a cup of dandelion tea.

BREAKFAST

Flax granola with approved fruit
OR
Smoothie with chia seeds and rye cracker with raw almond
butter (1 cracker for women, 3 for men)

LUNCH

Open-face vegetable sandwich with leftover mixed vegetables
topped with goat cheese and sunflower seeds
Spinach salad with apples
OR
Salad with leftover vegetables and goat cheese and rye cracker
with up to 6 tablespoons of Homemade Hummus (page 181;
1 cracker for women, 2 for men)

SNACK

Carrots with raw almond butter (1 to 2 tablespoons for women,
3 to 4 tablespoons for men)

DINNER

Approved protein (make sure to rotate)
2 cups of approved vegetables of choice (steamed, sautéed,
roasted, or grilled) and herbs of choice (make enough to have
some left over for dinner on Day Fourteen)
The Plan Chopped Salad (page 181) (be sure to make enough for
day 14)

DESSERT

1 ounce of dark chocolate or Cinnamon Poached Fruit (page 185)
with optional Katie's Whipped Coconut Cream (page 296)

WATER

Be sure to drink your recommended daily water intake throughout the day, ending by dinner.

Day Fourteen: Test New Breakfast Addition

UPON AWAKENING

- Weigh yourself and record the results in your Plan Journal.
- Drink 16 ounces of fresh water with lemon juice (after you weigh yourself).
- Take your liver support supplement and/or drink a cup of dandelion tea.

BREAKFAST

Test new breakfast item or test whole or lactose-free milk
Note: See page 132 for information on how to incorporate your favorite breakfast choices.

LUNCH

Leftover The Plan Chopped Salad with pumpkin seeds
1 apple or pear

SNACK

For women: 1 ounce of salt-free potato chips and ⅛ cup of Homemade Guacamole (page 204)
For men: 1½ ounces of salt-free potato chips and ¼ cup of Homemade Guacamole (page 204)

DINNER

Approved protein (make sure to rotate) on a bed of spinach and grated carrot
Leftover approved vegetables

DESSERT

1 ounce of dark chocolate or Cinnamon Poached Fruit (page 185) with optional Katie's Whipped Coconut Cream (page 296)

WATER

Be sure to drink your recommended daily water intake throughout the day, ending by dinner.

Day Fifteen: No Test

UPON AWAKENING

- Weigh yourself and record the results in your Plan Journal.
- Drink 16 ounces of fresh water with lemon juice (after you weigh yourself).
- Take your liver support supplement and/or drink a cup of dandelion tea.

BREAKFAST

Flax granola with approved fruit

OR

Flax granola mixed with approved cereal and fruit

LUNCH

Open-face sandwich with raw almond butter, sunflower seeds, and apple with mixed greens

OR

Any approved salad with 15 to 25 grams of vegetarian protein (no rice) and soup of choice (Butternut Squash Soup, page 182; Spicy Vegetarian, page 180; or Carrot Ginger, page 178)

Note: Please see page 131 for a list of vegetarian protein sources.

SNACK

1 to 2 cups of watermelon

DINNER

Chicken with Indian Spice rub (page 174; make enough to have 2 to 4 ounces left over for lunch on Day Sixteen)

Sautéed Kale with Vegetables (page 178; make enough to have some left over for lunch on Day Sixteen)

Steamed broccoli with lemon and Lemon Oil (page 176)

DESSERT

1 ounce of dark chocolate or Cinnamon Poached Fruit (page 185) with optional Katie's Whipped Coconut Cream (page 296)

WATER

Be sure to drink your recommended daily water intake throughout the day, ending by dinner.

Day Sixteen: Test Two Proteins in One Day

UPON AWAKENING

- Weigh yourself and record the results in your Plan Journal.
- Drink 16 ounces of fresh water with lemon juice (after you weigh yourself).
- Take your liver support supplement and/or drink a cup of dandelion tea.

BREAKFAST

Smoothie with 4 tablespoons of chia seeds and rye cracker with raw almond butter
OR
Bread with nut butter and approved fruit
OR
Flax granola mixed with approved cereal with approved fruit
OR
New approved breakfast

LUNCH

Leftover Sauteed Kale with Vegetables and chicken with Indian Spice Rub (2 ounces for women, 4 ounces for men)

1 apple

Note: Please pay attention to your energy levels in the afternoon today. If you notice a dip, then animal protein at lunch may not be ideal for you.

SNACK

Rye cracker with 1 ounce of cheese and apple slices (1 cracker for women, 3 crackers for men)

DINNER

Approved protein on a bed of mixed greens

Steamed, grilled, sautéed, or roasted approved vegetables with herbs of choice (make enough to have some left over for lunch on Day Seventeen)

DESSERT

1 ounce of dark chocolate or Cinnamon Poached Fruit (page 185) with optional Katie's Whipped Coconut Cream (page 296)

WATER

Be sure to drink your recommended daily water intake throughout the day, ending by dinner.

Day Seventeen: No Test

UPON AWAKENING

- Weigh yourself and record the results in your Plan Journal.
- Drink 16 ounces of fresh water with lemon juice (after you weigh yourself).
- Take your liver support supplement and/or drink a cup of dandelion tea.

BREAKFAST

Smoothie (page 174)
OR
Blueberry Compote (page 291; 1 cup for women, 1½ to 2 cups for men)

LUNCH

Leftover vegetables on a bed of spinach with sunflower and pumpkin seeds

SNACK

Carrots with Homemade Hummus (page 181) or raw almond butter

DINNER

Approved protein (make sure to rotate)
Vegetable Timbale (page 183; 1 cup for women, 2 cups for men; make enough to have some left over for lunch on Day Eighteen)
Mixed greens with carrot and apple (make enough to have some left over for lunch on Day Eighteen)

DESSERT

1 ounce of dark chocolate or Cinnamon Poached Fruit (page 185) with optional Katie's Whipped Coconut Cream (page 296)

WATER

Be sure to drink your recommended daily water intake throughout the day, ending by dinner.

Day Eighteen: Test New Restaurant (or New Vegetable)

UPON AWAKENING

- Weigh yourself and record the results in your Plan Journal.

- Drink 16 ounces of fresh water with lemon juice (after you weigh yourself).
- Take your liver support supplement and/or drink a cup of dandelion tea.

BREAKFAST

Flax granola mixed with approved cereal and fruit
OR
Smoothie with 4 tablespoons of chia seeds and rye cracker with raw almond butter (1 cracker for women, 3 crackers for men)
OR
New approved breakfast

LUNCH

Leftover mixed greens salad with Vegetable Timbale (1 cup for women, 2 cups for men) and pumpkin seeds

SNACK

For women: 1 ounce of salt-free potato chips and ⅛ cup of Homemade Guacamole (page 204; these are two foods high in potassium, which helps offset the sodium in restaurant food)
For men: 1½ ounces of salt-free potato chips and ¼ cup of Homemade Guacamole (page 204)

DINNER

Test a restaurant
Note: Please see page 142 for everything you need to know about testing restaurants.
OR
Any approved protein (make sure to rotate)
Any salad
Test any new (cooked) vegetable mixed with other approved vegetables

DESSERT

1 ounce of dark chocolate or Cinnamon Poached Fruit (page 185) with optional Katie's Whipped Coconut Cream (page 296) (or, if testing a new restaurant, please see page 141 for recommended dessert choices when dining out)

WATER

Be sure to drink your recommended daily water intake throughout the day, ending by dinner.

Day Nineteen: No Test

Repeat your favorite day with the most weight loss thus far.

Day Twenty: Test New Vegetable

UPON AWAKENING

- Weigh yourself and record the results in your Plan Journal.
- Drink 16 ounces of fresh water with lemon juice (after you weigh yourself).
- Take your liver support supplement and/or drink a cup of dandelion tea.

BREAKFAST

Flax granola with approved fruit
OR
Flax granola with approved cereal and approved fruit

LUNCH

Salad of choice with 15 to 25 grams of approved protein
Rye cracker with cheese and cucumber slices (1 cracker for women, 2 crackers for men)

SNACK

Approved fruit with a small handful of almonds

DINNER

Any approved protein (make sure to rotate)

Test a new vegetable and add to approved vegetables (can be steamed, sautéed, grilled, or roasted)

Arugula salad with pear and 1 tablespoon of grated Manchego cheese

DESSERT

1 ounce of dark chocolate or Cinnamon Poached Fruit (page 185) with optional Katie's Whipped Coconut Cream (page 296)

WATER

Be sure to drink your recommended daily water intake throughout the day, ending by dinner.

Thyroid Menu

The Thyroid Menu was specifically designed for people with thyroid issues. It creates a balance in the body to allow your thyroid to function optimally by omitting foods that are goitrogens. Goitrogens attack thyroid function, and while it is not an absolute that all goitrogens will affect you, there's a good chance they will. I've had people do wonderfully on spinach salad, and others gain 1.5 pounds and see their energy and BBT (basal body temperature) drop significantly. Besides avoiding potentially problematic goitrogenic foods, there are many other ways to help boost thyroid function, which you can read about in Part Two.

As with the regular menu, the first three days of The Plan's thyroid menu are a detox cleanse, which resets your body by decreasing inflammation and creating a purified, neutral base line against which you'll begin testing new foods. Days Four through Twenty are the testing phase, when we begin to systematically test foods, starting with the least reactive. I encourage you to read through Part Two for more insight into each phase, as well as answers to commonly asked questions, cooking tips, and more. For detailed information on each new food we test, please refer to the corresponding day in the regular menu listed in Part Two.

Note: Approved salad greens are baby romaine, red leaf, or green leaf lettuce. You can also download updated menus at www.lyngenet.com.

Day One: No Test

UPON AWAKENING

- Weigh yourself and record the results in your Plan Journal.
- Drink 16 ounces of fresh water with lemon juice (after you weigh yourself).
- Take your liver support supplement and/or drink a cup of dandelion tea along with your kelp and liquid B12 supplements (please refer to page 40 for more information about supplements for thyroid function).
- Take and record your basal body temperature (BBT) in your Plan Journal. Continue doing this until your temperature consistently reads above 97 degrees Fahrenheit, at which point you can taper off your supplements to a couple of times per week.

BREAKFAST

For women: 1 cup of flax granola (page 173) with ½ cup of blueberries
For men: 1½ cups of flax granola with 1 cup of blueberries
Silk coconut milk or Rice Dream

LUNCH

Carrot Ginger Soup (page 178) with sunflower seeds
Sautéed or steamed broccoli drizzled with Orange Oil (page 176) and lemon juice (make enough to have some left over for lunch on Day Two)
Baby romaine with ½ pear, ¼ avocado, and pumpkin seeds

SNACK

1 apple

DINNER

Sautéed Kale with Vegetables (page 178; make enough to have
some left over for dinner on Day Two) with Spicy Coco Sauce
(page 177)

Beet and Carrot Salad (page 178) with pumpkin seeds

WATER

Be sure to drink your recommended daily water intake throughout the day, ending by dinner.

Day Two: Almonds

UPON AWAKENING

- Weigh yourself and record the results in your Plan Journal.
- Drink 16 ounces of fresh water with lemon juice (after you
  weigh yourself).
- Take your liver support supplement and/or drink a cup of dandelion tea, along with your kelp and liquid B12 supplements
  (please refer to page 40 for more information about supplements for thyroid function).
- Take and record your BBT in your Plan Journal.

BREAKFAST

For women: 1 cup of flax granola with ½ cup of blueberries
For men: 1½ cups of flax granola with 1 cup of blueberries

LUNCH

Carrot Ginger Soup (page 178) with sunflower seeds
Baby romaine with ½ diced apple and ¼ avocado
Leftover sautéed or steamed broccoli with Orange Oil

SNACK

For women: ½ pear with a small handful of almonds

For men: 1 pear with a small handful of almonds

DINNER

For women: leftover Sautéed Kale with Vegetables with 1 cup of basmati rice with pumpkin seeds

For men: leftover Sautéed Kale with Vegetables with 2 cups of basmati rice

Beet and Carrot Salad (page 178) with sunflower seeds

WATER

Be sure to drink your recommended daily water intake through-out the day, ending by dinner.

Day Three: Chicken

UPON AWAKENING

- Weigh yourself and record the results in your Plan Journal.
- Drink 16 ounces of fresh water with lemon juice (after you weigh yourself).
- Take your liver support supplement and/or drink a cup of dandelion tea, along with your kelp and liquid B12 supplements (please refer to page 40 for more information about supplements for thyroid function).
- Take and record your BBT in your Plan Journal.

BREAKFAST

For women: 1 cup of flax granola with choice of ½ cup of blueberries or diced ½ pear

For men: 1½ cups of flax granola with choice of 1 cup of blueberries or 1 diced whole pear

LUNCH

Baby romaine with ¼ avocado, pumpkin seeds, and carrots
Cream of Broccoli Soup (page 294)

SNACK

Small handful of almonds *(if you tested reactive to almonds yesterday, you can replace this with an apple or pear)*

DINNER

Chicken with Italian Herbs and Orange Zest (page 182; 2 to 3 ounces for women, 4 ounces for men) on a bed of mixed greens
Roasted Italian Winter Vegetables (page 184; 1 to 2 cups for women, 2 to 3 cups for men; make enough to have some left over for lunch on Day Four)

WATER

Be sure to drink your recommended daily water intake throughout the day, ending by dinner.

Day Four: Cheese

Note: Please be sure to read "The Inside Scoop on Day Four" on page 99 so you don't miss out on all the fun stuff that Day Four reintroduces in addition to cheese, like coffee and wine!

UPON AWAKENING

- Weigh yourself and record the results in your Plan Journal.
- Drink 16 ounces of fresh water with lemon juice (after you weigh yourself).
- Take your liver support supplement and/or drink a cup of dandelion tea, along with your kelp and liquid B12 supplements (please refer to page 40 for more information about supplements for thyroid function).
- Take and record your BBT in your Plan Journal.

BREAKFAST

For women: 1 cup of flax granola with choice of approved fruit (½ cup of blueberries, ½ apple, or ½ pear)

For men: 1½ cups of flax granola with choice of approved fruit (1 cup of blueberries or 1 whole apple or pear)

LUNCH

Leftover Roasted Italian Winter Vegetables (1 cup for women, 2 cups for men) on a bed of baby romaine with pumpkin seeds and goat cheese (hard or soft)

SNACK

Carrots with raw almond butter (1 to 2 tablespoons for women, 3 to 4 tablespoons for men)

DINNER

Chicken with Mango Salsa (page 176)

Baby romaine with carrots and ¼ avocado (make enough to have some left over for lunch on Day Five)

Steamed or sautéed broccoli with Orange Oil (page 176) and chili flakes

DESSERT

1 ounce of dark chocolate or Cinnamon Poached Fruit (page 185) with optional Katie's Whipped Coconut Cream (page 296)

WATER

Be sure to drink your recommended daily water intake throughout the day, ending by dinner.

Note: This is a good time to retest for yeast. Check your tongue tomorrow morning to see if it has a white coating, which indicates a yeast overgrowth—especially if you include balsamic vinegar and wine in your menu today.

Day Five: Rye

UPON AWAKENING

- Weigh yourself and record the results in your Plan Journal.
- Drink 16 ounces of fresh water with lemon juice (after you weigh yourself).
- Take your liver support supplement and/or drink a cup of dandelion tea, along with your kelp and liquid B12 supplements (please refer to page 40 for more information about supplements for thyroid function).
- Take and record your BBT in your Plan Journal.

BREAKFAST

For women: 1 cup of flax granola with choice of approved fruit
For men: 1½ cups of flax granola with choice of approved fruit

LUNCH

Leftover dinner salad with goat cheese and sunflower seeds
Cream of Broccoli Soup (page 294)

SNACK

For women: 1 cracker with 1 to 2 tablespoons of raw almond butter and ½ apple
For men: 3 crackers with 3 to 4 tablespoons of raw almond butter and 1 whole apple

DINNER

Chicken with Spicy Apricot Glaze (page 177) on a bed of baby romaine
Sautéed, roasted, or grilled zucchini with onion and basil topped with Orange Oil (page 176) and 1 tablespoon grated Manchego
Beet and Carrot Salad (page 178) with sunflower seeds

DESSERT

1 ounce of dark chocolate or Cinnamon Poached Fruit (page 185) with optional Katie's Whipped Coconut Cream (page 296)

WATER

Be sure to drink your recommended daily water intake throughout the day, ending by dinner.

Day Six: Protein

UPON AWAKENING

- Weigh yourself and record the results in your Plan Journal.
- Drink 16 ounces of fresh water with lemon juice (after you weigh yourself).
- Take your liver support supplement and/or drink a cup of dandelion tea, along with your kelp and liquid B12 supplements (please refer to page 40 for more information about supplements for thyroid function).
- Take and record your BBT in your Plan Journal.

BREAKFAST

For women: 1 cup of flax granola with choice of approved fruit
For men: 1½ cups of flax granola with choice of approved fruit

LUNCH

Baby romaine with Beet and Carrot Salad (page 178), pumpkin seeds, and ¼ avocado
Rye cracker with goat cheese (1 cracker for women, 3 crackers for men)

SNACK

For women: ½ piece of approved fruit and a small handful of almonds

For men: 1 whole piece of approved fruit and a small handful of almonds

DINNER

Choose one protein from the list below to test on a bed of mixed greens:

Grilled *wild* white fish
Steak
Lamb
Venison
Duck
Egg

Roasted Squash, Kale, and Manchego Salad (page 179; make enough to have some left over for lunch on Day Seven)

Note: Please turn to page 105 to read more about the different animal protein sources and for cooking suggestions.

DESSERT

1 ounce of dark chocolate or Cinnamon Poached Fruit (page 185) with optional Katie's Whipped Coconut Cream (page 296)

WATER

Be sure to drink your recommended daily water intake throughout the day, ending by dinner.

Day Seven: Optional Test Chickpeas

UPON AWAKENING

- Weigh yourself and record the results in your Plan Journal.
- Drink 16 ounces of fresh water with lemon juice (after you weigh yourself).

- Take your liver support supplement and/or drink a cup of dandelion tea, along with your kelp and liquid B12 supplements (please refer to page 40 for more information about supplements for thyroid function).
- Take and record your BBT in your Plan Journal.

BREAKFAST

For women: 1 cup of flax granola with choice of approved fruit
For men: 1½ cups of flax granola with choice of approved fruit

LUNCH

Leftover Roasted Squash, Kale, and Manchego Salad with pumpkin seeds on a bed of baby romaine
Spicy Vegetarian Soup (page 180) if testing chickpeas

SNACK

Salt-free potato chips (1 ounce for women, 1½ ounces for men)
Note: Check out why salt-free potato chips are encouraged on The Plan on page 111.

DINNER

Chicken with Lemon Garlic Sauce (page 175) on a bed of mixed greens
Sautéed, grilled, or steamed vegetables (broccoli, carrots, zucchini, onions, and shiitakes) with garlic and herbs of choice (make enough to have some left over for dinner on Day Eight)

DESSERT

1 ounce of dark chocolate or Cinnamon Poached Fruit (page 185) with optional Katie's Whipped Coconut Cream (page 296)

WATER

Be sure to drink your recommended daily water intake throughout the day, ending by dinner.

Day Eight: Bread

UPON AWAKENING

- Weigh yourself and record the results in your Plan Journal.
- Drink 16 ounces of fresh water with lemon juice (after you weigh yourself).
- Take your liver support supplement and/or drink a cup of dandelion tea, along with your kelp and liquid B12 supplements (please refer to page 40 for more information about supplements for thyroid function).
- Take and record your BBT in your Plan Journal.

BREAKFAST

For women: 1 cup of flax granola with choice of approved fruit
For men: 1½ cups of flax granola with choice of approved fruit

LUNCH

1 slice of whole wheat or white bread with cheese, sunflower seeds, and avocado (2 slices of bread for men)

Note: Please do not use a multigrain bread; stick to plain white or wheat for this test. See page 116 for more information about bread.

Baby romaine and ½ diced apple

SNACK

Carrots with up to 6 tablespoons of Homemade Hummus only if testing chickpeas (page 181) or raw almond butter (1 to 2 tablespoons for women, 3 to 4 tablespoons for men)

DINNER

Protein that has been tested on a bed of baby romaine
Leftover vegetables from Day Seven's dinner

DESSERT

1 ounce of dark chocolate or Cinnamon Poached Fruit (page 185) with optional Katie's Whipped Coconut Cream (page 296)

WATER

Be sure to drink your recommended daily water intake throughout the day, ending by dinner.

Day Nine: Optional Test Chickpeas

UPON AWAKENING

- Weigh yourself and record the results in your Plan Journal.
- Drink 16 ounces of fresh water with lemon juice (after you weigh yourself).
- Take your liver support supplement and/or drink a cup of dandelion tea, along with your kelp and liquid B12 supplements (please refer to page 40 for more information about supplements for thyroid function).
- Take and record your BBT in your Plan Journal.

BREAKFAST

Flax granola with approved fruit

OR

For women: ¾ cup of cereal mixed with ¼ cup of flax granola and approved fruit

For men: 1½ cups of cereal mixed with ½ cup of flax granola and approved fruit

Note: Please avoid puffed rice cereals, as they impair digestion. For more information on rice cereal choices, see page 120.

OR

Bread with raw almond butter and approved fruit

LUNCH

Baby romaine with goat cheese, ¼ avocado, and sunflower seeds
Spicy Vegetarian Soup (page 180) if testing chickpeas

SNACK

The Plan Trail Mix (page 293; ¼ cup for women, ½ cup for men)

DINNER

Any approved protein (make sure to rotate)
Steamed or roasted winter squash (like butternut) with but-
    ter, cinnamon, and freshly ground black pepper (1 cup for
    women, 1 to 2 cups for men; make enough to have some left
    over for lunch on Day Ten)
The Plan Chopped Salad (page 181)

DESSERT

1 ounce of dark chocolate or Cinnamon Poached Fruit (page 185)
    with optional Katie's Whipped Coconut Cream (page 296)

WATER

Be sure to drink your recommended daily water intake through-
    out the day, ending by dinner.

Day Ten: Test New Protein

UPON AWAKENING

- Weigh yourself and record the results in your Plan Journal.
- Drink 16 ounces of fresh water with lemon juice (after you
  weigh yourself).
- Take your liver support supplement and/or drink a cup of dandelion tea, along with your kelp and liquid B12 supplements

(please refer to page 40 for more information about supplements for thyroid function).
- Take and record your BBT in your Plan Journal.

BREAKFAST

Flax granola with approved fruit
OR
Bread with nut butter and approved fruit

LUNCH

The Plan Chopped Salad (page 181) with pumpkin seeds
Leftover squash (1 cup for women, 1 to 2 cups for men) with
    1 tablespoon of grated Manchego

SNACK

Katie's Kale Chips (page 211) or salt-free potato chips (1 ounce
    for women, 1½ ounces for men)

DINNER

Choose one protein from the list below to test on a bed of mixed
    greens:

Grilled *wild* white fish
Steak
Lamb
Venison
Duck
Scallops
Pork
Cow's cheese
Lentils
Tempeh
Pinto beans
Egg

Sautéed kale with sunflower seeds, avocado, Lemon Oil (page 176), and goat cheese (make enough to have some left over for lunch on Day Eleven)

DESSERT

1 ounce of dark chocolate or Cinnamon Poached Fruit (page 185) with optional Katie's Whipped Coconut Cream (page 296)

WATER

Be sure to drink your recommended daily water intake throughout the day, ending by dinner.

Day Eleven: No Test

UPON AWAKENING

- Weigh yourself and record the results in your Plan Journal.
- Drink 16 ounces of fresh water with lemon juice (after you weigh yourself).
- Take your liver support supplement and/or drink a cup of dandelion tea, along with your kelp and liquid B12 supplements (please refer to page 40 for more information about supplements for thyroid function).
- Take and record your BBT in your Plan Journal.

BREAKFAST

Flax granola with approved fruit
OR
Blueberry Compote (page 291; 1 cup for women, 1½ to 2 cups for men)

LUNCH

Leftover sautéed kale with apple, avocado, sunflower and pumpkin seeds

SNACK

Carrots with up to 6 tablespoons of Homemade Hummus
(page 181) or raw almond butter (1 to 2 tablespoons for
women, 3 to 4 tablespoons for men)

DINNER

Any approved protein

Vegetable Timbale (page 183; 1 cup for women, 2 cups for men;
make enough to have some left over for lunch on Day Twelve)

Baby romaine salad

DESSERT

1 ounce of dark chocolate or Cinnamon Poached Fruit (page 185)
with optional Katie's Whipped Coconut Cream (page 296)

WATER

Be sure to drink your recommended daily water intake throughout the day, ending by dinner.

Day Twelve: Test New Vegetable

UPON AWAKENING

- Weigh yourself and record the results in your Plan Journal.
- Drink 16 ounces of fresh water with lemon juice (after you
  weigh yourself).
- Take your liver support supplement and/or drink a cup of dandelion tea, along with your kelp and liquid B12 supplements
  (please refer to page 40 for more information about supplements for thyroid function).
- Take and record your BBT in your Plan Journal.

BREAKFAST

Flax granola with approved fruit
OR
For women: ¾ cup of cereal mixed with ¼ cup of flax granola
and approved fruit
For men: 1½ cups of cereal mixed with ½ cup of flax granola and
approved fruit

LUNCH

Leftover Vegetable Timbale (1 cup for women, 2 cups for men)
and salad with pumpkin seeds
Rye cracker with raw almond butter (1 cracker for women, 3
crackers for men)

SNACK

The Plan Trail Mix (page 293) or potato chips

DINNER

Approved protein
Test a new vegetable mixed with other approved vegetables and
herbs of choice
*Note: We always test a new vegetable mixed in with other
approved vegetables to minimize the chance of reactivity. For
more on this and a list of lower-reactive vegetable choices,
please see page 129.*
Baby romaine with avocado and carrots

DESSERT

1 ounce of dark chocolate or Cinnamon Poached Fruit (page 185)
with optional Katie's Whipped Coconut Cream (page 296)

WATER

Be sure to drink your recommended daily water intake throughout the day, ending by dinner.

Day Thirteen: No Test

UPON AWAKENING

- Weigh yourself and record the results in your Plan Journal.
- Drink 16 ounces of fresh water with lemon juice (after you weigh yourself).
- Take your liver support supplement and/or drink a cup of dandelion tea, along with your kelp and liquid B12 supplements (please refer to page 40 for more information about supplements for thyroid function).
- Take and record your BBT in your Plan Journal.

BREAKFAST

Flax granola with approved fruit

OR

Smoothie (page 174) with chia seeds and rye cracker with raw almond butter (1 cracker for women, 3 crackers for men)

OR

For women: 1 cup of cereal mixed with 2 tablespoons of chia seeds and 1 ounce of sunflower seeds

For men: 2 cups of cereal mixed with 4 tablespoons of chia seeds and 1½ ounces of sunflower seeds

LUNCH

Open-face vegetable sandwich with leftover mixed vegetables topped with goat cheese

Baby romaine salad with sunflower seeds

OR

Approved salad with 15 to 25 grams of vegetarian protein (no rice) and soup of choice
Note: See page 131 for a list of vegetarian proteins.

SNACK

The Plan Trail Mix (page 293; ¼ cup for women, ½ cup for men)
OR
Katie's Kale Chips (page 211; 1 ounce for women, 1½ ounces for men)

DINNER

Approved protein on a bed of baby romaine with grated carrot (make enough to have some left over for dinner on Day Fourteen)
Grilled, steamed, or sautéed approved vegetables and herbs of choice (1 cup for women, 2 cups for men; make enough to have some left over for lunch on Day Fourteen)

DESSERT

1 ounce of dark chocolate or Cinnamon Poached Fruit (page 185) with optional Katie's Whipped Coconut Cream (page 296)

WATER

Be sure to drink your recommended daily water intake throughout the day, ending by dinner.

Day Fourteen: Test New Breakfast Addition

UPON AWAKENING

- Weigh yourself and record the results in your Plan Journal.
- Drink 16 ounces of fresh water with lemon juice (after you weigh yourself).
- Take your liver support supplement and/or drink a cup of dandelion tea, along with your kelp and liquid B12 supplements

(please refer to page 40 for more information about supplements for thyroid function).

- Take and record your BBT in your Plan Journal.

BREAKFAST

Test a new breakfast item or test whole or lactose-free milk
Note: See page 132 for information on how to incorporate your favorite breakfast choices.

LUNCH

Leftover vegetables (1 cup for women, 2 cups for men) on a bed of mixed greens with goat cheese
Rye cracker and up to 6 tablespoons of Homemade Hummus (page 181) (1 cracker for women, 3 crackers for men)

SNACK

Salt-free potato chips (1 ounce for women, 1½ ounces for men)

DINNER

Approved protein (make sure to rotate)
Leftover salad from Day Thirteen's dinner
Sautéed zucchini with basil, Lemon Oil (page 176), and 1 tablespoon of grated Manchego (make enough to have some left over for lunch on Day Fifteen)

DESSERT

1 ounce of dark chocolate or Cinnamon Poached Fruit (page 185) with optional Katie's Whipped Coconut Cream (page 296)

WATER

Be sure to drink your recommended daily water intake throughout the day, ending by dinner.

Day Fifteen: No Test

UPON AWAKENING

- Weigh yourself and record the results in your Plan Journal.
- Drink 16 ounces of fresh water with lemon juice (after you weigh yourself).
- Take your liver support supplement and/or drink a cup of dandelion tea, along with your kelp and liquid B12 supplements (please refer to page 40 for more information about supplements for thyroid function).
- Take and record your BBT in your Plan Journal.

BREAKFAST

Flax granola with approved fruit

OR

Blueberry Compote (page 291; 1 cup for women, 1½ to 2 cups for men)

LUNCH

Open-face sandwich with leftover zucchini, baby romaine, cheese, and sunflower seeds

1 whole approved fruit

OR

Any approved salad with 15 to 25 grams of vegetarian protein (no rice or chickpeas) and soup of choice (Butternut Squash, page 182; Spicy Vegetarian, page 180; or Carrot Ginger, page 178)

SNACK

Carrots with up to 6 tablespoons of Homemade Hummus (page 181)

DINNER

Chicken with Indian Spice Rub (page 174; make enough to have 2 to 4 ounces left over for lunch on Day Sixteen)

Sautéed Kale with Vegetables (page 178; make enough to have some left over for lunch on Day Sixteen)

Baby romaine with avocado

DESSERT

1 ounce of dark chocolate or Cinnamon Poached Fruit (page 185) with optional Katie's Whipped Coconut Cream (page 296)

WATER

Be sure to drink your recommended daily water intake throughout the day, ending by dinner.

Day Sixteen: Test Two Proteins

UPON AWAKENING

- Weigh yourself and record the results in your Plan Journal.
- Drink 16 ounces of fresh water with lemon juice (after you weigh yourself).
- Take your liver support supplement and/or drink a cup of dandelion tea, along with your kelp and liquid B12 supplements (please refer to page 40 for more information about supplements for thyroid function).
- Take and record your BBT in your Plan Journal.

BREAKFAST

Smoothie with 4 tablespoons of chia seeds and rye cracker with raw almond butter (1 cracker for women, 2 crackers for men)

OR

Bread with nut butter and approved fruit

OR

Flax granola mixed with approved cereal and fruit

OR
New approved breakfast

LUNCH

Leftover Sautéed Kale with Vegetables with chicken with Indian
Spice Rub (page 174; 2 ounces for women, 4 ounces for men)
½ apple
*Note: Please pay attention to your energy levels in the afternoon
today. If you notice a dip, then animal protein at lunch may
not be ideal for you.*

SNACK

For women: 1 rye cracker with cheese
For men: 3 rye crackers with cheese

DINNER

Approved protein on a bed of mixed greens
Steamed or sautéed approved vegetable

DESSERT

1 ounce of dark chocolate or Cinnamon Poached Fruit (page 185)
with optional Katie's Whipped Coconut Cream (page 296)

WATER

Be sure to drink your recommended daily water intake throughout the day, ending by dinner.

Day Seventeen: No Test

UPON AWAKENING

- Weigh yourself and record the results in your Plan Journal.
- Drink 16 ounces of fresh water with lemon juice (after you
  weigh yourself).

- Take you liver support supplement and/or drink a cup of dandelion tea, along with your kelp and liquid B12 supplements (please refer to page 40 for more information about supplements for thyroid function).
- Take and record your BBT in your Plan Journal.

BREAKFAST

Flax granola mixed with approved cereal and fruit

LUNCH

Spicy Chickpea Spinach Salad (page 180; make enough to have some left over for lunch on Day Eighteen)

Butternut Squash Soup (page 182)

Note: You can replace the spinach with baby romaine if you prefer. Please remember, however, that just because a food (like spinach) is a goitrogen, that doesn't mean it won't work for you. You know the rule: if you love it, test it!

SNACK

Rye cracker with raw almond butter (1 cracker for women, 3 crackers for men)

DINNER

Approved protein (make sure to rotate) on a bed of baby romaine

Vegetable Timbale (page 183; 1 cup for women, 2 cups for men; make enough to have some left over for lunch on Day Nineteen)

DESSERT

1 ounce of dark chocolate or Cinnamon Poached Fruit (page 185)
with optional Katie's Whipped Coconut Cream (page 296)

WATER

Be sure to drink your recommended daily water intake throughout the day, ending by dinner.

Day Eighteen: Test New Restaurant (or New Vegetable)

UPON AWAKENING

- Weigh yourself and record the results in your Plan Journal.
- Drink 16 ounces of fresh water with lemon juice (after you
  weigh yourself).
- Take your liver support supplement and/or drink a cup of dandelion tea, along with your kelp and liquid B12 supplements
  (please refer to page 40 for more information about supplements for thyroid function).
- Take and record your BBT in your Plan Journal.

BREAKFAST

Blueberry Compote (page 291) with sunflower seeds
OR
Smoothie with 4 tablespoons of chia seeds and rye cracker with
raw almond butter (1 cracker for women, 3 crackers for men)
OR
New approved breakfast

LUNCH

Leftover Spicy Chickpea Spinach Salad
Butternut Squash Soup (page 182)

SNACK

For women: 1 ounce of salt-free potato chips with ¼ cup of
Homemade Guacamole (page 204)

For men: 1 ounce of salt-free potato chips with ¼ cup of Homemade Guacamole (page 204; these are two foods high in
potassium, which helps offset the sodium in restaurant food)

DINNER

Test restaurant

*Note: Please see page 142 for everything you need to know about
testing restaurants.*

OR

Any approved protein

Any salad

Test any new (cooked) vegetable mixed with other approved vegetables

DESSERT

1 ounce of dark chocolate or Cinnamon Poached Fruit (page 185)
with optional Katie's Whipped Coconut Cream (page 296) or,
if testing a new restaurant, please see page 141 for recommended dessert choices when dining out

WATER

Be sure to drink your recommended daily water intake throughout the day, ending by dinner.

Day Nineteen: No Test

Repeat your favorite day thus far with the most weight loss.

Day Twenty: Test New Vegetable

UPON AWAKENING

- Weigh yourself and record the results in your Plan Journal.
- Drink 16 ounces of fresh water with lemon juice (after you weigh yourself).
- Take your liver support supplement and/or drink a cup of dandelion tea, along with your kelp and liquid B12 supplements (please refer to page 40 for more information about supplements for thyroid function).
- Take and record your BBT in your Plan Journal.

BREAKFAST

Flax granola with approved fruit
OR
Bread with raw almond butter and approved fruit
OR
New approved breakfast

LUNCH

Approved lunch with a minimum of 15 to 25 grams of vegetarian protein (no rice)
Choice of soup

SNACK

Katie's Kale Chips (page 211)

DINNER

Any approved protein (make sure to rotate)
Test a new vegetable and add to approved vegetables (can be steamed, sautéed, grilled, or roasted)
Baby romaine salad with pear slices

DESSERT

1 ounce of dark chocolate or Cinnamon Poached Fruit (page 185) with optional Katie's Whipped Coconut Cream (page 296)

WATER

Be sure to drink your recommended daily water intake throughout the day, ending by dinner.

The Five-Day Self-Test

This Five-Day Self-Test was created to give you a template for Days Twenty-One through Twenty-Five. Please be sure to refer to Chapter Six, which lays out the essential guidelines and instructions for testing on your own.

To begin, create a list of all the foods that have worked for you. These are the ones you'll plug into this template. On rest days, you'll stick to these entirely, and on test days, you'll eat them surrounding the new food or variable you are testing. Remember that you only want to test one new variable a day, so all the other foods you eat on test days should be friendly in order to give you the most accurate results.

Your daily menus should have one dense carbohydrate a day (like rice or bread) maximum and one animal protein a day maximum for weight loss (unless you tested well on two proteins in one day on Day Sixteen). For more information on the recommended frequency for including and rotating protein sources, please see Chapter Six. Most people do well when they moderate their intake of foods high in natural sugars, such as sweet potatoes, winter squashes, and roasted vegetables to twice a week. You'll find your own balance with all of these things in time.

Remember that protein is essential for weight loss. Women should aim to have 10 to 40 grams of protein for breakfast, 15 to 25 grams of protein for lunch, and 30 to 60 grams of protein for dinner each day. Men's daily consumption should be 15 to 60 grams of protein for breakfast, 20 to 40 grams of protein for lunch, and 45 to 70 grams of protein for dinner. Please see the sidebar on page 158 for a list of protein contents in animal and vegetarian sources.

Day 1: No Test

BREAKFAST

Any approved breakfast with 10 to 40 grams of approved protein for women (15 to 60 for men)

Approved fruit (½ piece for women, 1 whole piece for men)

LUNCH

Salad of choice with 15 to 25 grams of protein for women (20 to 40 for men)

Optional: add rye cracker for additional fiber (1 cracker for women, 2 crackers for men)

In winter, add approved soup or cooked vegetable of choice to enhance digestion

SNACK

Insert your favorite snack (please note that eating nuts too often may start to build nut sensitivity, so rotate your snacks)

DINNER

Approved protein of choice

Approved salad of choice

Approved cooked vegetable of choice

DESSERT

Approved dessert of choice

Day 2: Test Portion Size

Follow the guidelines for Day One to create a friendly menu, but test a larger portion of protein, dairy, or dense-grain carbohydrate.

Day 3: Test New Breakfast Item

BREAKFAST

Test a new breakfast item (whole milk, cereal, new fruit, etc. You can also test eggs; please note that if you do, and you choose animal protein for dinner, this will be a test for eggs and animal protein in one day.)

LUNCH

Approved salad of choice with 15 to 25 grams of protein for women (20 to 40 for men)

Optional: add rye cracker for additional fiber (1 cracker for women, 2 crackers for men)

In winter, add a soup or cooked vegetable of choice to enhance digestion

SNACK

Insert your favorite snack

DINNER

Approved protein of choice
Approved salad of choice
Approved cooked vegetable of choice

DESSERT

Approved dessert of choice

Day 4: Test Exercise

Repeat your best food day so far and test the variable of exercise to see how it affects weight loss.

Day 5: No Test

Repeat the guidelines for Day One.

New and Updated Recipes

BLUEBERRY COMPOTE—QUICK AND EASY VERSION

I don't know about you, but I don't have much time to prep. Or sit. Or let things gestate. So here's a quick version of my much-beloved blueberry pear compote.

2 cups blueberries
2¼ cups Silk coconut milk or Rice Dream
1 cup chia seeds
1 tbsp agave nectar
1 tsp vanilla extract
½ tsp cardamom
½ cup almond slivers or sunflower seeds

Combine all ingredients except almond slivers or sunflower seeds in small saucepan and bring to a boil.

Reduce heat and let simmer for 2 to 3 minutes, stirring constantly to prevent chia seeds from congealing.

Let sit for 5 minutes for a soft compote, or 10 minutes for a firmer compote.

Top with almond slivers or sunflower seeds. Serve warm.

Makes 4 servings.

COLUMBIA COUNTY FLAX GRANOLA

5¼ cups flaxseeds (brown and/or golden)
3 tbsp cinnamon
2¼ tbsp molasses
2¾ cups hot water

In a mixing bowl, stir together flaxseeds and cinnamon.

In a second, larger mixing bowl, thoroughly mix molasses into hot water (cool to room temperature).

Gradually pour and stir dry mixture into wet mixture. Stir until mixture begins to set. Cover bowl with lid or plastic wrap.

Let sit for 4 to 8 hours (best if kept refrigerated).

Preheat oven to 275 °F to 300 °F.

With a large mixing spoon, scoop mixture onto a parchment-covered cookie sheet. Use the flat of the spoon to spread the mix across the parchment, but not too firmly and not too thinly. Prepare additional cookie sheets with parchment as needed.

Bake for 20 minutes.

Remove cookie sheet(s) from oven. Gather edges of parchment together, then spread out again on cookie sheet and peel parchment away from granola—parchment should come off easily. If it sticks, bake for another 5 to 10 minutes, until parchment peels away from granola. Return cookie sheet(s) to oven for an additional 20 minutes.

Repeat 2 to 3 times, breaking up granola into clumps and clusters. The granola will gradually lose most of its moisture. When very little moisture is left, turn oven off and leave granola on sheet(s) in oven for 1 to 2 more hours.

Remove granola from oven, scoop into bowl, allow to fully cool, then stir in favorite add-ins: seeds, berries, etc.

Scoop granola mix into resealable bags. Store in a cool, dry place.

Makes 9 cups—more if you add fruit, seeds, etc.

THE PLAN TRAIL MIX

1 cup pumpkin seeds
¾ cup Craisins

Combine ingredients in plastic bag and shake. Store in airtight container or cool, dry place. Consume within a week.

Makes 6 to 8 servings.

CARROT SOUP ESSENCE—THE PLAN VEGAN SOUP STOCK

Even low-sodium vegetarian soup stocks are usually way too high in sodium. The magical carrot soup makes a great base for a soup stock, is more nutritious, and saves money!

2 tbsp extra virgin olive oil
2 cups chopped leeks (1 large)
1 large white onion, finely chopped
3 cloves garlic, minced
1 tbsp dried sage
1 tsp freshly ground black pepper
½ tsp sea salt
4 quarts Carrot Ginger Soup broth (page 295)
⅛ cup Low-Reactive Tomato Sauce (page 296)
½ cup chopped fresh parsley
1 bay leaf

In a large skillet, combine olive oil, leeks, onion, garlic, sage, pepper, and salt and sauté over medium heat for 2 to 3 minutes, until onion becomes translucent. In a medium-large soup pot, combine Carrot Ginger Soup broth, Low-Reactive Tomato Sauce, parsley, and bay leaf and bring to a boil. Add sautéed onion mixture. Let simmer for 20 minutes. Strain the soup essence, using a colander set over another pot. Use immediately or freeze in batches.

Makes 8 servings.

CREAM OF BROCCOLI SOUP

A protein-rich, delicious, and creamy soup that is a family favorite. Feel free to leave out the cayenne or Sriracha if you want to tone down the heat.

3 tbsp butter

1 large onion, chopped

1 tsp cumin

1 tbsp dried sage

½ tsp dried celery seed

2 cups low-sodium or homemade chicken broth, vegetable broth, or reserved Carrot Ginger Soup stock (page 295)

2 cups water

1 13- to 16-oz can full-fat unsweetened coconut milk

8 cups broccoli, chopped (about 4 heads broccoli)

4 cups zucchini, chopped (about 2 medium zucchini)

1 small cayenne pepper or 1 tbsp Sriracha sauce

1 medium avocado, peeled and pit removed

In a medium skillet, melt butter over medium heat. Add onion, cumin, sage, and celery seed and sauté until onion is tender. In a medium soup pot, combine broth, water, coconut milk, broccoli, zucchini, cayenne pepper or Sriracha, and sautéed onion. Bring to a boil, then simmer until vegetables are tender, about 30 minutes. Add avocado and puree in batches in blender or food processor.

Makes 6 to 8 servings.

CARROT GINGER SOUP

Carrot Ginger Soup, a mainstay of The Plan, is wonderfully anti-inflammatory and helps to rapidly restore GI balance after you eat a reactive food. This recipe, now updated, is for making the soup in bulk. This allows you to take advantage of those 5- and 10-lb bags of carrots on sale and to save time by freezing the excess for future use!

1 tbsp cinnamon
1 tbsp cumin
1 tbsp freshly ground black pepper
1 tsp cloves
1 tsp cardamom
½ tsp turmeric
½ tsp allspice
7 quarts water
2 tbsp extra virgin olive oil
5 lb carrots, chopped
2 large red onions, chopped
3 large zucchini, chopped
8 cloves garlic, peeled
5- to 6-inch piece fresh ginger, peeled

In a dry skillet, combine cinnamon, cumin, pepper, cloves, cardamom, turmeric, and allspice and toast the ground spices, stirring constantly, for 30 seconds. Put water in large soup pot. Add carrots, onions, zucchini, garlic, and ginger, then add toasted spices and extra virgin olive oil. Bring to a boil, then let simmer for 45 minutes, until carrots are soft. Reserve 2 quarts of liquid for future soups. Puree soup in batches in a blender or food processor.

Note: Add 1 can (13- to 16-oz) full-fat unsweetened coconut milk and 5 to 6 Vietnamese chili peppers for a creamier, spicier soup!

Makes 5 quarts, or 10 to 16 servings.

LOW-REACTIVE TOMATO SAUCE

1 bottle (24-oz) low-sodium tomato sauce
2½ cups Carrot Ginger Soup (page 178 and above)
1 garlic clove, minced
2 tbsp dried basil
1 tbsp dried oregano
½ tsp dried rosemary
Optional: Add 1 tbsp agave nectar or honey to make pizza sauce.

Combine all ingredients in large saucepan and simmer over low heat for 20 minutes. Let cool and pour into individual containers for freezing.

Makes 3 pints or 12 servings.

KATIE'S WHIPPED COCONUT CREAM

Our wonderful Dr. Katie, who works with us at The Plan, developed this dairy-free version of whipped cream so our lactose-intolerant friends don't have to miss out on a wonderful dessert topping.

1 can (13- to 16-oz) full-fat unsweetened coconut milk
Optional: 1 to 2 tbsp agave nectar
Optional: 1 tsp vanilla extract

Chill coconut milk in can for 8 hours or overnight.

Open can without shaking it. Separate cream on top from liquid and transfer to a large bowl; discard liquid. Add agave and vanilla to cream, if desired. Using a hand or stand mixer, whip coconut cream until it forms soft peaks, about 3 minutes. Serve immediately.

Makes 4 to 6 servings.

Acknowledgments

Writing this book has been a labor of love, and I could not have done it without support from the following people, to whom I am deeply indebted: Diana Baroni of Grand Central Publishing, Richard Pine of Inkwell Management, and Lesley Jane Seymour of *More* magazine. A special thanks to Debra Goldstein, whom I have driven crazy at times—okay, a *lot*—but who has been incredibly patient and truly a rock star.

The biggest hugs go to my clients, whom I love dearly, my staff, and my family. Thanks to you "Planners" for sharing your personal stories and triumphs and working so hard to find *your* path to health. You are truly an inspiration, and I never cease to be amazed by your strength.

Thank you to my incredibly strong, wonderful, and downright fun staff: Maggie Converse, truly my right hand; Cindy Hwang; Dr. Katie Reinholtz; and Dr. Lisa Boyer. Your work has helped to make The Plan what it is and allows us to help so many people. Thanks for all those concerned late-night and early-morning emails; you do this because you deeply care about healing.

Thank you, Bill Gillett, my fiancé, for keeping me sane and believing in me and this work, for cooking dinner, and for keeping our home together while I overwork! Thank you, dear Ted Recitas, for being a best friend, always ready to lend a helping hand. The biggest thanks goes to my beautiful son, Brayden. You kept asking when "the mommy book" would be finished so we could play more, but you always say with pride, "My mom makes people better."

Index

About the Author

LYN-GENET RECITAS has been studying holistic medicine for over thirty years. She started her practice working with immune response and hormonal balance twenty years ago on the West Coast and has been running health centers for the past ten years in New York and Westchester. Lyn-Genet and her team at The Plan have helped thousands of women and men over age thirty-five find easy, effective ways to lose weight, improve health, and reverse the aging process.